THE DR LI'S DIET COOKBOOK FOR BEGINNERS

Inspired by Dr. William Li

Nourishing, Easy Recipes to Boost Immunity, Fight Disease, and Heal Your Body Naturally

Irene A. Walker

Copyright © 2025 by [Irene A. Walker]
All rights reserved.

No part of this book may be reproduced, stored in a retrieval system, or transmitted in any form or by any means — electronic, mechanical, photocopying, recording, or otherwise — without the prior written permission of the copyright owner, except in the case of brief quotations embodied in critical reviews or articles.

This book is intended for informational purposes only. The author and publisher are not responsible for any adverse effects resulting from the use or application of the information contained herein. Always consult with a qualified healthcare professional before beginning any dietary, exercise, or health program.

Disclaimer

This cookbook is inspired by the nutritional principles promoted by Dr. William Li regarding the body's health defense systems. However, it is an independent work and is **not authored by, affiliated with, endorsed by, or sponsored by Dr. William Li, Dr. Li's organization, or any of his official programs**.

The recipes, meal plans, and tips provided in this book are intended for informational and educational purposes only and do not constitute medical advice.

Always seek the advice of a qualified healthcare professional before making changes to your diet or health routine. The author and publisher expressly disclaim all liability for any loss, damage, or injury caused or alleged to be caused directly or indirectly by the information in this book.

A Note to Readers

Dear Reader,

First, thank you so much for picking up this cookbook. It was truly created with your health, happiness, and kitchen confidence in mind.

While this book draws inspiration from the groundbreaking work of Dr. William Li and his research into how food can be used as powerful medicine, it is an independent project. This cookbook is not affiliated with, endorsed by, or connected to Dr. Li or his organization. Instead, it was lovingly written to help bring some of his key nutritional principles to life in an approachable, delicious, and budget-friendly way.

Think of this as your personal guide — packed with vibrant recipes, smart strategies, and a lot of heart — to making the science of healthy eating practical in your everyday life. Whether you're a beginner or already comfortable in the kitchen, I hope these pages inspire you to enjoy food in a way that nourishes not just your body, but your spirit too.

Wishing you health, joy, and many delicious meals,

[Irene A. Walker]

Contents

Copyright © 2025 by [Irene A. Walker] All rights reserved. 2

A Note to Readers 3

Introduction 7

Welcome to Food as Medicine 7

    Dr. Li's Five Defense Systems Explained 8

Chapter 1 10

Stocking Your Kitchen: Affordable Staples for Dr. Li's Diet 10

    Budget Tips: Saving on Berries, Nuts, and Seafood 12

    Tools for Easy Cooking 13

Chapter 2: Homemade Staples 14

    Chickpea Flour Tortillas (Gluten-free, microbiome-friendly) 14

    Almond-Oat Flatbread (Whole-grain, DNA protection) 16

    Buckwheat Pasta (Homemade, regeneration support) 17

    Cottage Cheese Herb Bread (Immunity-boosting) 19

    Avocado-Chickpea Pita (Heart-healthy) 20

    Maple-Walnut Granola (Angiogenesis support) 22

    Berry-Chia Jam (No added sugar, DNA protection) 23

    Cocoa-Hazelnut Spread (Regeneration-friendly dessert base) 24

    Coconut-Cashew Yogurt (Microbiome booster) 26

    Pumpkin Seed Crackers (Immunity and crunch) 27

Chapter 3: Angiogenesis Power (Balancing Blood Vessels 29

    Blueberry-Spinach Smoothie 29

    Tomato-Walnut Bruschetta 30

    Grilled Salmon with Raspberry Salsa ... 32

    Strawberry-Arugula Salad 33

    Green Tea Poached Chicken (Dinner, simple) 35

    Tuna-Stuffed Bell Peppers 36

    Cherry-Chia Pudding (Dessert, no sugar) 38

    Roasted Tomato Soup (Lunch, with basil) 39

    Pomegranate-Glazed Carrots (Side, vibrant) 41

    Blackberry-Cottage Cheese Toast (Snack) 42

    Beet Hummus (Snack, vibrant) 43

    Red Grape Sorbet (Dessert, no sugar) .. 44

    Tuna Quinoa Bowl (Lunch, omega-3s) . 45

    Kale-Avocado Breakfast Bowl (Breakfast, regeneration) 46

    Shiitake and Spinach Soup (Dinner, immunity) 47

    Turmeric-Ginger Roasted Cauliflower Steaks (Dinner, DNA protection) 48

    Garlic-Herb Roasted Chickpeas (Snack, microbiome) 49

    Oyster Mushroom Tacos (Dinner, gut-friendly) 50

Berry-Coconut Popsicles (Dessert, DNA protection) 51
Banana-Oat Muffins (Breakfast, microbiome) 52

Chapter 4: Regeneration Boost (Stem Cell Support) 54

Dark Chocolate-Oat Bites (Snack, No Sugar) 54
Olive Oil Poached Cod (Dinner, Mediterranean) 55
Sweet Potato and Kale Hash (Lunch, Hearty) 56
Cocoa-Banana Smoothie (Breakfast, quick) 57
Spinach and Mushroom Frittata 58
Fig and Almond Tart (Dessert, whole-grain crust) 59
Lentil-Pumpkin Stew (Dinner, cozy) 60
Apple-Walnut Salad 61
Roasted Parsnips with Thyme 62
Almond Butter Cups 62
Kale Chips 63
(Snack, crunchy and light) 63
Golden Turmeric Quinoa 64
Zucchini Ribbon Salad with Lemon-Pepper Dressing 65
Sweet Potato and Black Bean Tacos 66

Chapter 5: Hearty and Healthy Comfort Foods 68

Wild Mushroom Stir Fry 68
Baked Sweet Potato with Tahini Drizzle 69
Turmeric Chicken Skillet 71
Grilled Salmon with Broccoli Salsa 72
Lentil & Eggplant Shepherd's Pie 74
Cauliflower Steaks with Pesto 75
Black Garlic Roasted Chicken 77
Bok Choy & Tofu Stir Fry 78

Chapter 6: DNA Defense 80
(Anti-Cancer and Anti-Aging) 80

Broccoli-Avocado Salad 81
Grilled Mackerel with Citrus 83
Cauliflower Steaks with Tahini 84
Cinnamon-Roasted Pears 86
Brussels Sprouts with Pomegranate 87
Chickpea Patties with Spinach 88
Orange-Zest Chia Pudding 90
Cabbage and Apple Stir-Fry 91
Turmeric Tea Latte 92
Roasted Radishes with Garlic (Side, vibrant) 93
Citrus Sorbet (Dessert, no sugar) 94
Creamy Broccoli Soup (Lunch, heart-healthy) 95
Lentil-Walnut Salad (Lunch, protein-packed) 96
Baked Cod with Tomato-Olive Relish ... 97

Chapter 7: Immunity Warriors (Fighting Infections) 99

Ginger-Turmeric Tea 99
Garlic & Lemon Chicken Soup 100
Spinach and Kale Power Salad 101

- Elderberry Syrup Smoothie 102
- Miso Soup with Seaweed and Tofu 103
- Citrus and Berry Smoothie 104
- Fermented Kimchi with Brown Rice ... 105
- Roasted Garlic and Broccoli 106
- Chia Seed Pudding with Turmeric and Honey 107
- Carrot & Ginger Immunity Juice 108
- Chicken and Mushroom Stir Fry 108
- Apple Cider Vinegar Detox Drink 109
- Roasted Butternut Squash Soup 110
- Zinc-Rich Pumpkin Seed Pesto 111
- Lentil & Tomato Soup with Spinach ... 112
- Tips for Success 113

Chapter 8: 30 Day Meal Plan 117
- shopping list 121
- How to Stick to Dr. Li's Diet Without Feeling Overwhelmed 123
- Favorite Meal Prep Hacks for Dr. Li's Diet 125
- 20 burning questions and answers for beginners 126

Introduction

Welcome to Food as Medicine

What if the secret to a healthier, longer life was already in your kitchen? Imagine sitting down to a vibrant bowl of blueberry-spinach salad or a warm slice of homemade chickpea tortilla stuffed with roasted veggies, knowing each bite is actively fighting disease, boosting your energy, and protecting your future. This isn't a fantasy—it's the power of *food as medicine*, a revolutionary approach championed by Dr. William W. Li, world-renowned physician, scientist, and author of *Eat to Beat Disease*. Welcome to *Dr. Li's Diet Cookbook*, your guide to turning everyday ingredients into delicious meals that supercharge your body's natural defenses.

You don't need a medical degree or a pantry stocked with exotic ingredients to eat like Dr. Li. You *do* need simple, clean, and affordable recipes that make sense for your busy life—recipes that taste as good as they feel. That's exactly what this book delivers: tasty dishes inspired by Dr. Li's groundbreaking research, crafted to be accessible, budget-friendly, and packed with flavor. No processed sugars, no white flour, no hard-to-find "superfoods" you've never heard of. Instead, you'll find pantry staples like oats, canned chickpeas, and frozen berries transformed into meals that support your health without breaking the bank or your schedule.

Why food as medicine? Because your body is a powerhouse, equipped with five natural defense systems—angiogenesis, regeneration, microbiome, DNA protection, and immunity—that can prevent and even reverse diseases like cancer, heart disease, and diabetes. Dr. Li's research shows that specific foods, from kale to salmon to dark chocolate, activate these systems like a conductor leading an orchestra. Every recipe in this book is designed to harness that power, with clear explanations of *why* each dish works. Whether you're a health enthusiast, a busy parent, or someone looking to feel better without restrictive diets, this cookbook is your roadmap to eating smarter, not harder.

But let's be real: you've probably bought cookbooks before, only to find recipes that call for ingredients you can't pronounce or techniques that belong on a cooking show. We heard you—loud and clear. Readers of other "healthy" cookbooks have been let down by processed ingredients, expensive grocery lists, or recipes that don't live up to the hype. That's why we've gone back to the basics, focusing on whole foods, homemade staples (like almond-oat bread and chickpea tortillas), and trendy favorites like avocado and cottage cheese. Each recipe is tested for simplicity (think 15–30 minutes) and affordability, with tips for sourcing ingredients at your local supermarket. This isn't just a cookbook; it's a promise that healthy eating can be delicious, doable, and deeply rewarding.

Picture this: In just 15 minutes, you're savoring a bowl of garlic-mushroom soup that's not only comforting but also boosting your immunity to fight off colds. Or imagine your family raving about a no-sugar berry-chia pudding that's secretly protecting their DNA from aging. That's the magic of this book—meals that heal while they delight. Ready to unlock your kitchen's potential? Let's dive into the science that makes it possible, inspired by Dr. Li's vision for a healthier world.

Dr. Li's Five Defense Systems Explained

At the heart of Dr. William W. Li's food-as-medicine philosophy lies a simple but profound truth: your body is built to protect itself, and the right foods can amplify that protection. Through decades of research, Dr. Li identified five health defense systems that act like an internal security team, working 24/7 to keep you thriving. These systems—angiogenesis, regeneration, microbiome, DNA protection, and immunity—are the foundation of this cookbook, and every recipe is crafted to support one or more of them. Here's a closer look at how they work and why food is their secret weapon.

- **Angiogenesis: Balancing Blood Vessels**
Your body relies on blood vessels to deliver oxygen and nutrients, but too many or too few can fuel diseases like cancer or heart disease. Angiogenesis is your body's ability to grow or prune blood vessels as needed. Foods like blueberries, tomatoes, and green tea contain compounds that inhibit excess vessel growth (starving tumors) or promote healthy circulation. Try our *Grilled Salmon with Raspberry Salsa* to see how delicious angiogenesis support can be.

- **Regeneration: Renewing Your Cells**
Your body is constantly rebuilding itself, thanks to stem cells that repair tissues and organs. Foods like kale, olive oil, and dark chocolate provide nutrients that fuel this regeneration, helping you recover from injury, slow aging, and stay vibrant. Our *Kale-Avocado Breakfast Bowl* is a morning boost that keeps your cells in top shape.

- **Microbiome: Nurturing Your Gut**
Your gut is home to trillions of bacteria that influence digestion, mood, and immunity. A healthy microbiome fights inflammation and disease, and foods like yogurt, chickpeas, and fermented veggies feed the good bacteria. Dive into our *Chickpea-Avocado Lettuce Wraps* for a gut-loving lunch that's as trendy as it is tasty.

- **DNA Protection: Shielding Your Genes**
Your DNA is under constant attack from stress, pollution, and aging, but certain foods act like bodyguards, repairing damage and preventing mutations that lead to cancer or chronic illness. Cruciferous veggies (like broccoli), citrus fruits, and turmeric are DNA defenders. Our *Turmeric-Ginger Roasted Cauliflower Steaks* make protection a weeknight favorite.

- **Immunity: Fighting Infections**
  Your immune system is your first line of defense against viruses, bacteria, and even cancer cells. Foods like garlic, mushrooms, and berries supercharge your immune response, keeping you resilient. Our *Shiitake and Spinach Soup* is a cozy way to arm your body against invaders.

Why It Matters: Dr. Li's research, featured in his bestselling book *Eat to Beat Disease* and his viral TED Talk, shows that these systems don't work in isolation—they collaborate like a symphony. Eating a variety of whole foods amplifies their effects, creating a cascade of health benefits. This cookbook translates that science into 100 recipes, from breakfast smoothies to hearty dinners, each labeled with the defense systems it supports. You'll know exactly how your *Cinnamon-Roasted Pears* are protecting your DNA or how your *Garlic-Herb Roasted Chickpeas* are boosting immunity.

You don't have to overhaul your life to eat like Dr. Li. With recipes that take 5–10 ingredients and minimal prep, you'll be amazed at how easy it is to turn science into supper. Whether you want to prevent disease, boost energy, or simply feel your best, this book is your invitation to a healthier you—one delicious bite at a time.

Chapter 1

Stocking Your Kitchen: Affordable Staples for Dr. Li's Diet

One of the biggest secrets to successfully following Dr. Li's diet is preparation. When your kitchen is filled with real, healing foods, making nourishing meals becomes second nature. You don't need expensive gadgets, trendy health foods, or hard-to-find ingredients. You simply need a smart foundation: everyday, affordable staples that work hard to protect your health.

Pantry Staples

The pantry is your first line of defense. Stock it with nutrient-dense basics that can turn into quick breakfasts, lunches, dinners, or snacks. Whole grains like brown rice, quinoa, old-fashioned oats, and even barley are essential. They provide fiber, energy, and support your gut microbiome — key pillars of Dr. Li's anti-disease philosophy.

Keep a good supply of canned or dried beans like lentils, chickpeas, black beans, and cannellini beans. If you prefer convenience, low-sodium canned versions are perfect — just rinse them before using to reduce any extra salt.

Flours like almond flour, oat flour, or whole wheat flour are excellent for baking healthy breads, pancakes, or coatings for fish and chicken. Choose minimally processed options when possible.

Nuts and seeds such as almonds, walnuts, chia seeds, flaxseeds, and pumpkin seeds are powerhouse foods. A small handful daily offers healthy fats, protein, and critical plant compounds. Store them in your freezer to keep them fresh longer.

For cooking, stick to extra virgin olive oil and avocado oil. Avoid vegetable oils and blends, which are often heavily processed. A few types of vinegar — apple cider, balsamic, and red wine vinegar — add brightness to meals without piling on calories.

Canned wild-caught salmon, sardines, and coconut milk are practical staples for quick meals rich in healthy fats and protein. Herbs and spices like turmeric, cumin, cinnamon, oregano, garlic powder, and rosemary will add flavor and health benefits to your dishes without needing lots of salt or sugar.

When you need a touch of sweetness, use natural options like raw honey or pure maple syrup, and only in moderation. For condiments, keep simple options like salt-free mustard, tamari (a gluten-free alternative to soy sauce), and tahini, a nutrient-rich sesame paste.

Fridge and Freezer Staples

A well-stocked fridge keeps fresh, vibrant ingredients ready at your fingertips.

Fill it with colorful vegetables like broccoli, spinach, kale, carrots, zucchini, sweet potatoes, tomatoes, and cucumbers. Buying seasonal produce saves money and ensures the best flavor and nutrition. Fresh fruits like blueberries, apples, oranges, lemons, avocados, and bananas support immunity and provide essential antioxidants.

Keep a small amount of organic, free-range chicken breast and wild-caught fish such as salmon, sardines, or cod. These clean proteins form the 20% of your diet that's animal-based, following Dr. Li's guidelines.

Plant-based milks like unsweetened almond or oat milk are great alternatives to dairy. Always check labels to avoid hidden sugars and unnecessary additives.

You might also want to include organic tofu or tempeh if you enjoy plant proteins — both are now easy to find in most supermarkets.

Your freezer is your backup plan. Keep frozen vegetables like broccoli, spinach, edamame, peas, and cauliflower rice on hand. Frozen fruits like berries and mango chunks are perfect for quick smoothies or healthy desserts. Frozen produce is picked at peak ripeness and flash-frozen, locking in nutrition, so don't hesitate to use it!

Basic Prep Tools You'll Need

You don't need a gourmet kitchen to succeed.

A few essential tools will carry you through every recipe:

- A sharp chef's knife
- A sturdy cutting board
- A good blender (for smoothies, soups, and dressings)
- A quality skillet (preferably cast iron or stainless steel)
- A baking sheet for roasting
- A medium and a large saucepan
- Measuring cups and spoons
- A mixing bowl

With these simple tools, you can prepare every recipe in this book easily, without needing fancy appliances.

Smart Budget Tips

You can make healthy eating more affordable with a few simple tricks:

- Buy dry beans and lentils instead of canned — they cost less and yield more.
- Choose store-brand versions of oats, rice, oil, and vinegars.
- Stock up on frozen vegetables and fruits when they're on sale.
- Shop farmers' markets late in the day — vendors often discount produce they don't want to haul home.

You don't need to spend a fortune to stock a healing kitchen. You simply need to choose **real foods, smartly and consistently.**

Budget Tips: Saving on Berries, Nuts, and Seafood

Eating for health doesn't mean you have to spend a fortune. Some of the most powerful foods in Dr. Li's diet — berries, nuts, and seafood — can feel pricey at first glance. But with a little strategy, you can enjoy these superfoods without straining your wallet.

Berries: Buy Smart and Freeze

Fresh berries like blueberries, strawberries, and raspberries are nutritional goldmines. But buying them fresh all the time can get expensive, especially when they're out of season.

One of the smartest tricks is to buy **frozen organic berries**. Frozen berries are picked at peak ripeness and flash-frozen, preserving all their nutrients — and they often cost half as much as fresh ones.

If you prefer fresh berries, shop seasonally. When berries are in season locally, prices drop dramatically. Buy extra and freeze them yourself for later smoothies, baking, or toppings.

Another tip: Check farmers' markets toward the end of the day. Farmers often discount berries they don't want to haul home.

Nuts: Shop in Bulk and Store Wisely

Nuts like almonds, walnuts, and cashews are essential in Dr. Li's approach for their healthy fats and cancer-fighting properties. Buying nuts in small packages can drain your budget fast.

Instead, **buy in bulk** from warehouse clubs, health food stores, or even online. Look for sales and store brands — there's often no real difference in quality, just a lower price tag.

When you bring them home, store nuts in the **freezer** to keep them fresh for months. This prevents them from going rancid and wasting your money.

You can also rotate: buy a different type of nut each month (almonds one month, walnuts the next) to spread out the cost while still getting variety.

Seafood: Prioritize Frozen and Canned

Wild-caught salmon, sardines, and cod are stars of Dr. Li's clean animal protein approach.
Fresh seafood can be costly, but the frozen section is your best friend.

Frozen wild-caught salmon fillets are often cheaper than fresh, and they cook beautifully straight from frozen if needed. Canned wild-caught salmon and sardines are another budget-friendly option — they're packed with omega-3s, easy to store, and quick to use in salads, patties, or simple dinners.

Look for sales and stock up when prices drop.
Buying a few extra cans of salmon or

sardines when they're on sale is an easy way to stretch your dollar without sacrificing nutrition.

Tools for Easy Cooking

You don't need a fancy kitchen or professional chef's setup to eat like Dr. Li recommends.

A few basic tools — many of which you might already own — will make healthy cooking quicker, easier, and much more enjoyable.

1. A Good Knife

A sharp chef's knife is your number one tool. It makes chopping vegetables, fruits, fish, and chicken faster, safer, and more efficient. Invest in one good knife and keep it sharpened — it will transform your cooking.

2. Cutting Boards

Have at least two cutting boards: one for produce, and one for meat and fish. This helps avoid cross-contamination and makes cleanup easier. Wooden or heavy plastic boards are easiest to work with and clean.

3. Blender or Food Processor

For smoothies, creamy soups, dressings, and nut butters, a basic blender is essential. If you want to take it a step further, a food processor can chop, grind, and blend almost anything quickly — but it's optional for beginners.

4. Quality Skillet

A heavy-bottomed stainless steel or cast-iron skillet is perfect for quick sautés, stir-fries, and searing fish or chicken. Non-stick pans work too but look for safer, non-toxic coatings if possible.

5. Baking Sheets and Pans

Roasting vegetables and fish is one of the easiest healthy cooking methods. One or two sturdy baking sheets will serve you well. Also keep a basic loaf pan for baking simple breads or healthy desserts.

6. Saucepan and Stockpot

You'll need a medium-sized saucepan for simmering grains, soups, and sauces, and a larger pot for making broths or bigger batches of food.

7. Measuring Cups and Spoons

Precision matters when baking and helps you get comfortable with new recipes. Pick up a set of dry measuring cups, a liquid measuring cup, and a set of measuring spoons — nothing fancy needed.

8. Mixing Bowls

A few sturdy mixing bowls make it easy to toss salads, marinate fish, mix batters, and prep ingredients.

Chapter 2: Homemade Staples

Chickpea Flour Tortillas (Gluten-free, microbiome-friendly)

Prep Time: 5 minutes
Cooking Time: 12 minutes
Total Time: 17 minutes
Servings: 4 (8 tortillas, 2 per serving)

Nutritional Information (per serving, 2 tortillas):

- Calories: 180 kcal
- Protein: 7 g
- Fat: 6 g (1 g saturated)
- Carbohydrates: 24 g (4 g fiber, 0 g added sugar)
- Sodium: 300 mg
- Key Nutrients: Iron (10% DV), Magnesium (8% DV), Folate (12% DV)

Ingredients:

- 1 cup chickpea flour (also called garbanzo bean flour or besan)
- 1 cup water
- 1 tablespoon olive oil (extra-virgin preferred for flavor)
- ½ teaspoon salt
- ½ teaspoon dried oregano or cumin (optional, for flavor)
- Cooking spray or 1 teaspoon olive oil (for skillet)

Instructions:

- **Prepare the Batter**: In a medium mixing bowl, combine chickpea flour, salt, and optional oregano or cumin. Whisk to break up any lumps. Slowly pour in the water and olive oil, whisking continuously until the batter is smooth and slightly thinner than pancake batter. Let the batter rest for 5 minutes to hydrate the flour, which helps the tortillas hold together.

- **Heat the Skillet**: Place a non-stick skillet over medium heat. Lightly coat with cooking spray or brush with 1 teaspoon olive oil to prevent sticking. Let the skillet heat for 1–2 minutes until hot (a drop of water should sizzle).

- **Cook the Tortillas**: Stir the batter once more. Pour ¼ cup of batter into the center of the skillet, tilting and swirling the pan to spread it into a thin, 6-inch circle. (If the batter is too thick, add 1 tablespoon water to thin it.) Cook for 1–2 minutes until the edges lift slightly and the bottom is golden with brown spots. Gently flip with a spatula and cook the other side for 1 minute until golden. Transfer to a plate and cover with a clean kitchen towel to keep warm.

- **Repeat**: Repeat with the remaining batter, stirring the batter before each tortilla to prevent settling. Adjust heat to medium-low if the skillet gets too hot, and reapply cooking spray or oil as needed. You should get 8 tortillas total.

- **Serve or Store**: Serve warm as wraps for *Chickpea-Avocado Lettuce Wraps*, tacos with grilled veggies, or as a side for dipping in hummus. Store leftovers in an airtight container in the fridge for up to 3 days or freeze (separated by parchment paper) for up to 1 month. Reheat in a skillet or microwave for 10–15 seconds.

Substitutions:

- **Chickpea Flour**: No direct substitute, as it's key for texture and nutrition. Find it in the gluten-free or international aisle of supermarkets, or at Indian grocery stores (labeled besan).

- **Olive Oil**: Avocado oil or melted coconut oil works.

- **Oregano/Cumin**: Skip or use any dried herb/spice you have (e.g., paprika, thyme).

- **Water**: Unsweetened almond milk adds a subtle nutty flavor but isn't necessary.

Why it Works:
Chickpea flour is a microbiome superstar, rich in prebiotic fiber that feeds beneficial gut bacteria, supporting digestion, immunity, and even mood, as Dr. William W. Li highlights in *Eat to Beat Disease*. Its high protein and iron content also promote regeneration, helping your body repair tissues. Olive oil adds heart-healthy monounsaturated fats that support angiogenesis balance, ensuring proper blood vessel growth. Unlike store-bought tortillas, which often contain refined flour and additives, these homemade versions are clean, gluten-free, and packed with nutrients that align with Dr. Li's food-as-medicine philosophy. The optional spices like oregano or cumin enhance flavor while adding anti-inflammatory compounds, making every bite a step toward better health.

Serving Suggestion: Pair with *Tomato-Walnut Bruschetta* for a microbiome- and angiogenesis-boosting meal, or use as a base for *Oyster Mushroom Tacos* to double down on gut-friendly fiber.

Almond-Oat Flatbread (Whole-grain, DNA protection)

Prep Time: 10 minutes
Cooking Time: 15 minutes
Total Time: 25 minutes
Servings: 4 (4 flatbreads, 1 per serving)

Nutritional Information (per serving, 1 flatbread):

- Calories: 200 kcal
- Protein: 6 g
- Fat: 12 g (1 g saturated)
- Carbohydrates: 18 g (4 g fiber, 0 g added sugar)
- Sodium: 150 mg
- Key Nutrients: Vitamin E (15% DV), Magnesium (10% DV), Fiber (16% DV)
  Note: Nutritional values are approximate, based on USDA data. Adjust for specific brands or Substitutions.

Ingredients:

- 1 cup almond flour
- ¾ cup rolled oats (gluten-free if needed)
- ½ cup water
- 1 tablespoon olive oil
- ½ teaspoon baking powder
- ¼ teaspoon salt
- 1 teaspoon dried rosemary (optional, for flavor)
- Cooking spray or 1 teaspoon olive oil (for skillet)

Instructions:

- **Blend the Oats**: In a food processor or blender, pulse rolled oats until they form a fine flour (about 30 seconds). This creates a whole-grain base that's easy to digest.
- **Mix the Dough**: In a medium mixing bowl, combine oat flour, almond flour, baking powder, salt, and optional rosemary. Stir in water and olive oil until a soft, slightly sticky dough forms. If too dry, add 1 tablespoon water; if too wet, add 1 tablespoon almond flour. Knead gently in the bowl for 30 seconds to combine.
- **Shape the Flatbreads**: Divide the dough into 4 equal balls. Place each ball on a piece of parchment paper and flatten with your hands or a rolling pin into a 6-inch round, about ¼-inch thick. Smooth edges with your fingers for a neat shape.
- **Cook the Flatbreads**: Heat a non-stick skillet over medium heat and lightly coat with cooking spray or 1 teaspoon olive oil. Cook one flatbread at a time for 2–3 minutes per side, until golden brown and slightly crisp. Alternatively, bake all 4 flatbreads on a parchment-lined baking sheet at 375°F (190°C) for 12–15 minutes, flipping halfway, until golden.
- **Serve or Store**: Serve warm with *Tomato-Walnut Bruschetta* (page XX) or as a wrap for grilled veggies. Store

leftovers in an airtight container in the fridge for up to 4 days or freeze (separated by parchment) for up to 1 month. Reheat in a skillet or toaster oven for 1–2 minutes.

Substitutions:

- **Almond Flour**: Hazelnut flour works, but avoid coconut flour (it's too absorbent).
- **Rolled Oats**: Quick oats are fine; ensure gluten-free if needed.
- **Olive Oil**: Avocado oil or melted butter (for non-vegan) can substitute.
- **Rosemary**: Skip or use any dried herb (e.g., oregano, basil).

Why it Works: Almond flour and oats are rich in vitamin E and fiber, which Dr. Li highlights in *Eat to Beat Disease* for their DNA-protective properties, neutralizing free radicals that cause cellular damage and aging. Oats also provide beta-glucans, supporting gut health and immunity, while olive oil's monounsaturated fats promote balanced angiogenesis. This flatbread is a whole-grain, gluten-free alternative to processed breads, delivering nutrients that shield your genes and support overall wellness, perfectly aligned with Dr. Li's clean-eating principles.

Serving Suggestion: Top with *Avocado-Chickpea Pita* for lunch, or serve with *Roasted Tomato Soup* for a cozy meal.

Buckwheat Pasta (Homemade, regeneration support)

Prep Time: 20 minutes
Cooking Time: 5 minutes
Total Time: 35 minutes
Servings: 4 (about 1 cup cooked pasta per serving)

Nutritional Information (per serving, 1 cup cooked):

- Calories: 170 kcal
- Protein: 6 g
- Fat: 2 g (0 g saturated)
- Carbohydrates: 34 g (3 g fiber, 0 g added sugar)
- Sodium: 150 mg
- Key Nutrients: Magnesium (12% DV), Manganese (20% DV), Niacin (8% DV

Ingredients:

- 1 cup buckwheat flour (plus extra for dusting)
- ½ cup whole wheat flour (or gluten-free all-purpose flour for gluten-free)
- ¾ cup water (adjust as needed)
- Pinch of salt (optional)

Instructions:

- **Make the Dough**: In a medium mixing bowl, combine buckwheat flour, whole wheat flour, and salt (if using). Gradually add water, stirring with a fork until a shaggy dough forms. Knead on a lightly floured surface for 3–5 minutes until smooth and elastic. If too sticky, add 1 tablespoon buckwheat flour; if too dry, add 1 teaspoon water.

- **Roll the Dough**: Divide the dough into 2 equal portions. On a floured surface, roll one portion into a thin rectangle, about 1/16-inch thick (like a lasagna sheet). Dust with buckwheat flour to prevent sticking. Repeat with the second portion.

- **Cut the Pasta**: Lightly flour the dough surface, then fold loosely and slice into ¼-inch wide strips for fettuccine or 1-inch for pappardelle. Unfold the strips and dust with a little buckwheat flour to keep them from sticking.

- **Cook the Pasta**: Bring a large pot of water to a boil and add a pinch of salt. Add the pasta and cook for 3–5 minutes, stirring occasionally, until al dente (tender but with a slight bite). Taste a strand to check doneness. Drain with a slotted spoon or colander.

- **Serve or Store**: Toss with olive oil and *Kale and Mushroom Frittata* (page XX) sauce or a simple garlic-herb oil. Store uncooked pasta in an airtight container in the fridge for up to 2 days or freeze for up to 1 month. Cooked pasta keeps in the fridge for 3 days; reheat with a splash of water to revive.

Substitutions:

- **Buckwheat Flour**: No direct substitute, but quinoa flour can work (adjust water as it's drier). Find buckwheat flour in health food aisles or online.

- **Whole Wheat Flour**: Use all-purpose flour or gluten-free blend for gluten-free; avoid oat flour (too soft).

- **Water**: Unsweetened almond milk can add subtle flavor.

Why it Works: Buckwheat is a regeneration powerhouse, rich in flavonoids and magnesium that Dr. Li notes in *Eat to Beat Disease* support stem cell activity, aiding tissue repair and recovery. Its fiber also promotes microbiome health, while whole wheat flour (or gluten-free alternative) adds complex carbs for sustained energy. This pasta skips refined flours, delivering a nutrient-dense, clean-eating option that supports your body's natural renewal processes, perfectly aligned with Dr. Li's principles.

Serving Suggestion: Pair with *Spinach and Mushroom Frittata* for a regeneration-focused dinner, or toss with *Turmeric-Ginger Sauce* for added DNA protection.

Cottage Cheese Herb Bread (Immunity-boosting)

Prep Time: 15 minutes
Cooking Time: 40 minutes
Total Time: 55 minutes
Servings: 8 (1 slice per serving, 1 loaf)

Nutritional Information (per serving, 1 slice):

- Calories: 160 kcal
- Protein: 8 g
- Fat: 5 g (1 g saturated)
- Carbohydrates: 21 g (3 g fiber, 1 g sugar)
- Sodium: 250 mg
- Key Nutrients: Calcium (10% DV), Vitamin B12 (8% DV), Selenium (12% DV)

Ingredients:

- 1 cup cottage cheese (low-fat or full-fat)
- 1 ½ cups whole wheat flour (or gluten-free all-purpose flour)
- ½ cup almond flour
- 2 large eggs
- 2 tablespoons olive oil
- 1 teaspoon baking powder
- ½ teaspoon baking soda
- ½ teaspoon salt
- 1 teaspoon minced garlic (or ½ teaspoon garlic powder)
- 1 tablespoon chopped fresh dill or parsley (or 1 teaspoon dried)

Instructions:

- **Preheat Oven**: Preheat your oven to 350°F (175°C). Line an 8x4-inch loaf pan with parchment paper or lightly grease with olive oil.
- **Blend Wet Ingredients**: In a food processor or blender, combine cottage cheese, eggs, olive oil, and minced garlic. Blend until smooth, about 30 seconds, to create a creamy base.
- **Mix Dry Ingredients**: In a large mixing bowl, whisk together whole wheat flour, almond flour, baking powder, baking soda, salt, and fresh dill or parsley.
- **Combine and Form Dough**: Pour the wet mixture into the dry ingredients and stir with a spatula until just combined, forming a thick batter. Avoid overmixing to keep the bread tender. If too dry, add 1 tablespoon water.
- **Bake the Bread**: Transfer the batter to the prepared loaf pan, smoothing the top with a spatula. Bake for 35–40 minutes, until golden brown and a toothpick inserted in the center comes out clean. Let cool in the pan for 10 minutes, then transfer to a wire rack to cool completely.
- **Serve or Store**: Slice and serve with *Shiitake and Spinach Soup* (page XX) or as a sandwich base with avocado. Store in an airtight container in the fridge for up

to 5 days or freeze slices for up to 1 month. Reheat in a toaster oven or microwave for 10–15 seconds.

Substitutions:

- **Cottage Cheese**: Greek yogurt (plain, unsweetened) works but may be tangier.

- **Whole Wheat Flour**: Use all-purpose or gluten-free blend for gluten-free.

- **Almond Flour**: Oat flour or hazelnut flour can substitute.

- **Eggs**: Flax eggs (1 tbsp ground flax + 3 tbsp water per egg) for vegan, but texture may be denser.

- **Fresh Herbs**: Use dried herbs (reduce to 1 tsp) or skip.

Why it Works:
Cottage cheese is rich in probiotics and protein, which Dr. Li notes in *Eat to Beat Disease* support immunity by enhancing gut health and immune cell function. Garlic's allicin compounds have antimicrobial properties, further boosting infection resistance. Whole wheat and almond flours provide fiber and antioxidants for DNA protection, while olive oil supports angiogenesis balance. This bread is a clean, immunity-boosting alternative to processed loaves, delivering trendy cottage cheese in a form that aligns with Dr. Li's principles.

Serving Suggestion: Use as a base for *Cottage Cheese Veggie Dip* or pair with *Citrus-Avocado Salad* for an immunity- and DNA-protective meal.

Avocado-Chickpea Pita (Heart-healthy)

Prep Time: 15 minutes
Cooking Time: 0 minutes
Total Time: 15 minutes
Servings: 4 (1 pita half per serving)

Nutritional Information (per serving, 1 pita half):

- Calories: 250 kcal

- Protein: 8 g

- Fat: 10 g (1.5 g saturated)

- Carbohydrates: 34 g (7 g fiber, 2 g sugar)

- Sodium: 320 mg

- Key Nutrients: Folate (15% DV), Vitamin K (20% DV), Potassium (12% DV) *Note*: Nutritional values are approximate, based on USDA data. Adjust for specific brands or Substitutions.

Ingredients:

- 1 cup canned chickpeas, rinsed and drained

- 1 ripe avocado, pitted and peeled

- 1 tablespoon lemon juice

- 1 tablespoon olive oil

- ½ teaspoon ground cumin

- ¼ teaspoon salt

- 2 whole wheat pita breads (or *Almond-Oat Flatbread*, page XX), halved
- 1 cup baby spinach or arugula
- ½ cup shredded carrot
- ¼ cup thinly sliced red onion

Instructions:

- **Mash the Filling**: In a medium mixing bowl, combine chickpeas, avocado, lemon juice, olive oil, cumin, and salt. Mash with a fork or potato masher until mostly smooth with some chunky texture, similar to guacamole. Taste and adjust seasoning with more lemon juice or salt if desired.
- **Prepare the Pita**: If using store-bought pita, warm briefly in a toaster oven or microwave for 10 seconds to soften. Carefully open each pita half to create a pocket. If using *Almond-Oat Flatbread*, fold gently to hold fillings.
- **Assemble the Pita**: Stuff each pita half with ¼ of the chickpea-avocado mixture (about ⅓ cup). Add a layer of spinach or arugula, followed by shredded carrot and red onion. Press gently to pack the fillings.
- **Serve or Store**: Serve immediately with a side of *Cucumber-Tomato Salad* (page XX) or cut into wedges for a snack. Store leftover filling in an airtight container in the fridge for up to 2 days; assemble pitas just before eating to prevent sogginess.

Substitutions:

- **Chickpeas**: White beans or lentils work well.
- **Avocado**: Mashed Greek yogurt or hummus for a lower-fat option, though less heart-healthy.
- **Whole Wheat Pita**: Use gluten-free pita or lettuce wraps for gluten-free.
- **Spinach/Arugula**: Any leafy green (e.g., kale, romaine).
- **Lemon Juice**: Lime juice or apple cider vinegar.

Why it Works: Chickpeas are rich in fiber and prebiotics, feeding beneficial gut bacteria that Dr. Li links to heart health and microbiome balance in *Eat to Beat Disease*. Avocado's monounsaturated fats lower bad cholesterol and support angiogenesis, promoting healthy blood vessels. Olive oil and leafy greens add anti-inflammatory compounds, while cumin provides antioxidants. This pita is a heart-healthy, clean-eating powerhouse that avoids processed ingredients, aligning with Dr. Li's principles and delivering trendy ingredients readers love.

Serving Suggestion: Pair with *Berry-Chia Jam* on *Cottage Cheese Herb Bread* for a heart- and immunity-boosting meal.

Maple-Walnut Granola (Angiogenesis support)

Prep Time: 5 minutes
Cooking Time: 25 minutes
Total Time: 30 minutes
Servings: 8 (½ cup per serving)

Nutritional Information (per serving, ½ cup):

- Calories: 220 kcal
- Protein: 5 g
- Fat: 14 g (1.5 g saturated)
- Carbohydrates: 20 g (4 g fiber, 6 g sugar)
- Sodium: 75 mg
- Key Nutrients: Omega-3s (10% DV), Magnesium (15% DV), Vitamin E (8% DV)

Ingredients:

- 2 cups rolled oats (gluten-free if needed)
- 1 cup walnuts, roughly chopped
- ¼ cup pure maple syrup
- 2 tablespoons olive oil
- 1 teaspoon vanilla extract
- ½ teaspoon ground cinnamon
- ¼ teaspoon salt

Instructions:

- **Preheat Oven**: Preheat your oven to 325°F (165°C). Line a baking sheet with parchment paper to prevent sticking.
- **Mix Ingredients**: In a large mixing bowl, combine oats, walnuts, cinnamon, and salt. In a small bowl, whisk together maple syrup, olive oil, and vanilla extract. Pour the wet mixture over the dry ingredients and stir until evenly coated.
- **Spread and Bake**: Spread the granola mixture in an even layer on the prepared baking sheet. Bake for 20–25 minutes, stirring halfway with a spatula, until golden brown and fragrant. The granola will crisp up as it cools.
- **Cool and Break**: Remove from the oven and let cool completely on the baking sheet (about 15 minutes) to form clusters. Break into desired chunk sizes.
- **Serve or Store**: Serve over *Coconut-Cashew Yogurt* (page XX) or with fresh berries. Store in an airtight container at room temperature for up to 2 weeks or freeze for up to 2 months.

Substitutions:

- **Walnuts**: Pecans or almonds work well.
- **Maple Syrup**: Honey or agave nectar, though maple is preferred for flavor.
- **Olive Oil**: Coconut oil or avocado oil.
- **Oats**: Use certified gluten-free oats for gluten-free diets.

Why it Works: Walnuts are a star in Dr. Li's angiogenesis research, containing ellagic acid and omega-3s that inhibit excess blood vessel growth, starving tumors and supporting heart health, as noted in *Eat to Beat Disease*. Oats provide fiber for microbiome health, while maple syrup offers natural sweetness with trace minerals, avoiding processed sugars. Olive oil's monounsaturated fats further promote vascular health. This granola is a clean, angiogenesis-supporting snack that's both delicious and aligned with Dr. Li's principles.

Serving Suggestion: Sprinkle over *Blueberry-Spinach Smoothie* bowl for a double dose of angiogenesis support, or pair with *Berry-Chia Jam*

Berry-Chia Jam (No added sugar, DNA protection)

Prep Time: 5 minutes
Cooking Time: 10 minutes
Total Time: 15 minutes
Servings: 8 (2 tablespoons per serving, about 1 cup total)

Nutritional Information (per serving, 2 tablespoons):

- Calories: 40 kcal
- Protein: 1 g
- Fat: 2 g (0 g saturated)
- Carbohydrates: 6 g (3 g fiber, 2 g sugar)
- Sodium: 0 mg

- Key Nutrients: Vitamin C (10% DV), Manganese (8% DV), Antioxidants (anthocyanins)

Note: Nutritional values are approximate, based on USDA data. Adjust for specific brands.

Ingredients:

- 2 cups mixed berries (fresh or frozen; e.g., strawberries, blueberries, raspberries)
- 2 tablespoons chia seeds
- 2 tablespoons water
- 1 tablespoon lemon juice
- 1 teaspoon vanilla extract (optional, for depth)

Instructions:

- **Cook the Berries**: In a small saucepan, combine berries, water, and lemon juice over medium heat. Cook for 5–7 minutes, stirring occasionally, until berries break down and release juices. Mash gently with a wooden spoon for a smoother texture or leave chunkier if preferred.

- **Add Chia Seeds**: Stir in chia seeds and vanilla extract (if using). Reduce heat to low and simmer for 2–3 minutes, stirring constantly, until the mixture thickens slightly. The chia seeds will absorb liquid and create a jam-like consistency.

- **Cool and Set**: Remove from heat and let cool for 5 minutes. The jam will continue to thicken as it cools. Transfer to a clean glass jar or airtight container.

- **Serve or Store**: Serve warm or chilled on *Cottage Cheese Herb Bread* (page XX) or as a topping for *Maple-Walnut Granola* (page XX). Store in the fridge for up to 1 week or freeze for up to 3 months.

Substitutions:

- **Mixed Berries**: Use any single berry (e.g., all blueberries) or cherries.
- **Chia Seeds**: Ground flaxseeds can work but may alter texture slightly.
- **Lemon Juice**: Lime juice or orange juice for a different citrus note.
- **Water**: Increase to 3 tablespoons if using fresh berries for extra liquid.

Why it Works: Berries are Dr. Li's go-to for DNA protection, loaded with anthocyanins and vitamin C that neutralize free radicals, preventing cellular damage and aging, as highlighted in *Eat to Beat Disease*. Chia seeds add omega-3s and fiber, supporting microbiome health and heart health via angiogenesis balance. This jam skips added sugars, using berries' natural sweetness for a clean, DNA-protective spread that aligns with Dr. Li's principles and satisfies the demand for no-sugar recipes.

Serving Suggestion: Spread on *Almond-Oat Flatbread* with *Coconut-Cashew Yogurt* for a DNA- breakfast.

Cocoa-Hazelnut Spread (Regeneration-friendly dessert base)

Prep Time: 10 minutes
Cooking Time: 5 minutes (for toasting hazelnuts)
Total Time: 15 minutes
Servings: 8 (2 tablespoons per serving, about 1 cup total)

Nutritional Information (per serving, 2 tablespoons):

- Calories: 140 kcal
- Protein: 3 g
- Fat: 12 g (1 g saturated)
- Carbohydrates: 7 g (2 g fiber, 4 g sugar)
- Sodium: 40 mg
- Key Nutrients: Vitamin E (10% DV), Magnesium (8% DV), Antioxidants (flavonoids)
  Note: Nutritional values are approximate, based on USDA data. Adjust for specific brands or Substitutions.

Ingredients:

- 1 cup hazelnuts (skinless or skin-on)

- 2 tablespoons unsweetened cocoa powder (preferably dark, 70%+ cacao)
- 3 tablespoons pure maple syrup
- 2 tablespoons olive oil
- ¼ cup water (adjust for consistency)
- ¼ teaspoon salt
- ½ teaspoon vanilla extract (optional, for depth)

Instructions:

- **Toast the Hazelnuts**: Preheat your oven to 350°F (175°C). Spread hazelnuts on a baking sheet and toast for 5–7 minutes, until fragrant and lightly golden. Shake the pan halfway to ensure even toasting. Let cool for 5 minutes. If using skin-on hazelnuts, rub them in a clean kitchen towel to remove most skins (some bits are fine).
- **Blend the Spread**: In a food processor or high-powered blender, process toasted hazelnuts for 2–3 minutes, scraping down the sides as needed, until they form a smooth nut butter. Add cocoa powder, maple syrup, olive oil, salt, and vanilla extract (if using). Blend for another 1–2 minutes, gradually adding water 1 tablespoon at a time, until the spread is creamy and spreadable. Adjust water for desired thickness.
- **Taste and Adjust**: Taste the spread and add more maple syrup for sweetness or cocoa for richer flavor, blending briefly to combine.
- **Serve or Store**: Transfer to a glass jar or airtight container. Serve as a spread on *Cottage Cheese Herb Bread* (page XX), a dip for apple slices, or a swirl in *Coconut-Cashew Yogurt* (page XX). Store in the fridge for up to 2 weeks; stir before using as oil may separate.

Substitutions:

- **Hazelnuts**: Almonds or cashews work, but hazelnuts pair best with cocoa.
- **Maple Syrup**: Honey or agave nectar for similar sweetness.
- **Olive Oil**: Avocado oil or melted coconut oil.
- **Cocoa Powder**: Carob powder for a caffeine-free option, though flavor differs.
- **Water**: Unsweetened almond milk for a creamier texture.

Why it Works: Hazelnuts are rich in vitamin E and magnesium, which Dr. Li highlights in *Eat to Beat Disease* for supporting stem cell activity and tissue regeneration, aiding recovery and vitality. Unsweetened cocoa powder provides flavonoids that protect DNA and promote angiogenesis balance, inhibiting harmful blood vessel growth. Maple syrup offers natural sweetness with trace minerals, avoiding processed sugars, while olive oil's monounsaturated fats support heart health. This spread is a regeneration-friendly dessert base that's clean, nutrient-dense, and aligned with Dr. Li's principles.

Serving Suggestion: Spread on *Buckwheat Pasta* for a dessert-inspired dish or pair with *Berry-Chia Jam* for a regeneration- and DNA-protective treat.

Coconut-Cashew Yogurt (Microbiome booster)

Prep Time: 10 minutes
Cooking Time: 0 minutes (plus 12–24 hours fermentation)
Total Time: 10 minutes active, 12–24 hours total
Servings: 6 (½ cup per serving, about 3 cups total)

Nutritional Information (per serving, ½ cup):

- Calories: 180 kcal
- Protein: 3 g
- Fat: 16 g (10 g saturated)
- Carbohydrates: 8 g (2 g fiber, 2 g sugar)
- Sodium: 30 mg
- Key Nutrients: Probiotics, Magnesium (10% DV), Copper (8% DV)
  Note: Nutritional values are approximate, based on USDA data. Adjust for specific brands.

Ingredients:

- 1 can (13.5 oz) full-fat coconut milk
- ½ cup raw cashews, soaked in water for 4 hours and drained
- 2 tablespoons maple syrup (or honey)
- 1 probiotic capsule (or ¼ cup plain, unsweetened store-bought yogurt with live cultures)
- 1 teaspoon vanilla extract (optional, for flavor)
- 2 tablespoons water (for blending)

Instructions:

- **Blend the Base**: In a high-powered blender, combine coconut milk, soaked cashews, maple syrup, vanilla extract (if using), and water. Blend on high for 1–2 minutes until completely smooth and creamy, scraping down sides as needed.
- **Add Probiotics**: Pour the mixture into a clean glass jar or bowl. Open the probiotic capsule and sprinkle the powder (or add store-bought yogurt) into the mixture. Stir gently with a wooden or plastic spoon (avoid metal, as it can interfere with fermentation).
- **Ferment**: Cover the jar with cheesecloth or a clean kitchen towel and secure with a rubber band. Place in a warm, draft-free spot (e.g., on a counter or in an off oven) for 12–24 hours. Taste after 12 hours; it should be tangy. Longer fermentation (up to 24 hours) increases tanginess.
- **Chill and Serve**: Once fermented, stir the yogurt, cover with a lid, and refrigerate for at least 4 hours to thicken and chill. Serve with *Maple-Walnut Granola* (page XX) or as a base for smoothies. Store in the fridge for up to 1 week.

Substitutions:

- **Coconut Milk**: Use lite coconut milk for lower fat, but texture may be thinner.
- **Cashews**: Almonds or macadamia nuts, soaked similarly.
- **Maple Syrup**: Omit for unsweetened yogurt or use agave nectar.
- **Probiotic Capsule**: Plain, unsweetened kefir (2 tbsp) can work.

Why it Works: Coconut milk and cashews provide healthy fats and prebiotic fiber, feeding beneficial gut bacteria that Dr. Li links to microbiome health in *Eat to Beat Disease*. Probiotics from the capsule or yogurt starter enhance gut diversity, supporting immunity and reducing inflammation. Maple syrup adds minimal sweetness with trace minerals, avoiding processed sugars. This yogurt is a clean, microbiome-boosting staple that's trendy and aligned with Dr. Li's principles, perfect for gut health enthusiasts.

Serving Suggestion: Top with *Berry-Chia Jam* and fresh fruit for a microbiome- and DNA-protective breakfast.

Pumpkin Seed Crackers (Immunity and crunch)

Prep Time: 10 minutes
Cooking Time: 20 minutes
Total Time: 30 minutes
Servings: 6 (8 crackers per serving, about 48 crackers total)

Nutritional Information (per serving, 8 crackers):

- Calories: 150 kcal
- Protein: 5 g
- Fat: 12 g (1.5 g saturated)
- Carbohydrates: 6 g (3 g fiber, 0 g sugar)
- Sodium: 100 mg
- Key Nutrients: Zinc (15% DV), Omega-3s (10% DV), Iron (8% DV)
  Note: Nutritional values are approximate, based on USDA data. Adjust for specific brands.

Ingredients:

- 1 cup raw pumpkin seeds (pepitas)
- ¼ cup ground flaxseeds
- ½ cup water
- 2 tablespoons olive oil
- ½ teaspoon smoked paprika
- ¼ teaspoon salt

- ¼ teaspoon garlic powder (optional, for flavor)

Instructions:

- **Preheat Oven**: Preheat your oven to 350°F (175°C). Line a baking sheet with parchment paper.

- **Process Seeds**: In a food processor or blender, pulse pumpkin seeds until coarsely ground (like coarse sand), about 10–15 seconds. This ensures a crunchy but cohesive texture.

- **Mix Dough**: In a medium mixing bowl, combine ground pumpkin seeds, ground flaxseeds, smoked paprika, salt, and garlic powder (if using). Add water and olive oil, stirring until a thick, sticky dough forms. Let sit for 5 minutes to allow flaxseeds to absorb water.

- **Shape Crackers**: Place the dough between two sheets of parchment paper and roll to ⅛-inch thickness (about a 10x12-inch rectangle). Remove the top parchment and transfer the bottom parchment with dough to the baking sheet. Use a knife or pizza cutter to score into 1-inch squares or rectangles (for 48 crackers).

- **Bake**: Bake for 18–20 minutes, until edges are golden and crisp. If centers are soft, bake an additional 2–3 minutes. Let cool completely on the baking sheet (about 10 minutes) to crisp further, then break along score lines.

- **Serve or Store**: Serve with *Coconut-Cashew Yogurt* (page XX) as a dip or top with sliced veggies. Store in an airtight container at room temperature for up to 2 weeks.

Substitutions:

- **Pumpkin Seeds**: Sunflower seeds or sesame seeds work.

- **Flaxseeds**: Chia seeds can substitute, though texture may be slightly gummier.

- **Olive Oil**: Avocado oil or melted coconut oil.

- **Smoked Paprika**: Chili powder or cumin for a different flavor.

Why it Works: Pumpkin seeds are rich in zinc and magnesium, which Dr. Li notes in *Eat to Beat Disease* support immune cell function and infection resistance. Flaxseeds provide omega-3s and fiber, promoting microbiome health and angiogenesis balance. Olive oil's monounsaturated fats further support heart health. These crackers are a clean, gluten-free, immunity-boosting snack that avoids processed ingredients, delivering crunch and nutrition in line with Dr. Li's principles.

Serving Suggestion: Pair with *Tomato-Walnut Bruschetta* for an immunity- and angiogenesis-supporting appetizer.

Chapter 3: Angiogenesis Power (Balancing Blood Vessels

Blueberry-Spinach Smoothie

Prep Time: 5 minutes
Cooking Time: 0 minutes
Total Time: 5 minutes
Servings: 2 (1 cup per serving, about 2 cups total)

Nutritional Information (per serving, 1 cup):

- Calories: 180 kcal
- Protein: 4 g
- Fat: 10 g (1 g saturated)
- Carbohydrates: 20 g (5 g fiber, 10 g sugar)
- Sodium: 50 mg
- Key Nutrients: Vitamin C (15% DV), Vitamin K (30% DV), Antioxidants (anthocyanins)

Ingredients:

- 1 cup frozen blueberries
- 1 cup fresh baby spinach (or frozen, thawed)
- ½ ripe avocado, pitted and peeled
- 1 tablespoon almond butter
- 1 cup unsweetened almond milk
- 1 teaspoon lemon juice
- ½ teaspoon ground cinnamon (optional, for warmth)

Instructions:

- **Blend the Smoothie**: In a blender, combine frozen blueberries, spinach, avocado, almond butter, almond milk, lemon juice, and cinnamon (if using). Blend on high for 30–60 seconds until smooth and creamy, scraping down the sides if needed. If too thick, add 1–2 tablespoons more almond milk; if too thin, add a few more blueberries.
- **Taste and Adjust**: Taste the smoothie and adjust with more lemon juice for brightness or almond butter for richness, blending briefly to combine.
- **Serve**: Pour into two glasses or reusable bottles for an on-the-go breakfast. Serve immediately for the freshest flavor, or chill for up to 4 hours.
- **Store**: If not consuming right away, store in an airtight container in the fridge for up to 24 hours. Shake or stir before drinking, as separation is natural.

Substitutions:

- **Blueberries**: Frozen mixed berries or cherries work well.
- **Spinach**: Kale or arugula, though kale may need more blending.
- **Avocado**: ¼ cup Greek yogurt or ½ banana for creaminess.

- **Almond Butter**: Peanut butter or cashew butter.
- **Almond Milk**: Any unsweetened plant-based milk (e.g., oat, soy) or water.

Why it Works: Blueberries are a cornerstone of Dr. Li's angiogenesis research in *Eat to Beat Disease*, rich in anthocyanins that inhibit harmful blood vessel growth, starving tumors and supporting heart health. Spinach provides vitamin K and folate for DNA protection, while avocado and almond butter offer healthy fats that promote microbiome health and satiety. This smoothie is a clean, no-added-sugar breakfast that aligns with Dr. Li's principles, delivering trendy ingredients in a quick, nutrient-dense package.

Serving Suggestion: Pair with *Maple-Walnut Granola* sprinkled on top for a crunchy, angiogenesis-boosting breakfast bowl.

Tomato-Walnut Bruschetta

Prep Time: 15 minutes
Cooking Time: 0 minutes
Total Time: 15 minutes
Servings: 4 (2 pieces per serving, 8 pieces total)

Nutritional Information (per serving, 2 pieces):

- Calories: 160 kcal
- Protein: 4 g
- Fat: 10 g (1 g saturated)
- Carbohydrates: 14 g (3 g fiber, 2 g sugar)
- Sodium: 200 mg
- Key Nutrients: Lycopene (antioxidants), Omega-3s (8% DV), Vitamin C (12% DV)

Ingredients:

- 2 cups cherry tomatoes, halved
- ¼ cup walnuts, finely chopped
- 2 tablespoons olive oil
- 1 tablespoon balsamic vinegar
- 1 teaspoon fresh basil, chopped (or ½ teaspoon dried)
- ¼ teaspoon salt
- ⅛ teaspoon black pepper
- 4 slices *Almond-Oat Flatbread* (page XX) or whole-grain bread, toasted

Instructions:

- **Prepare the Topping**: In a medium mixing bowl, combine cherry tomatoes, chopped walnuts, olive oil, balsamic vinegar, basil, salt, and pepper. Toss gently to coat. Let sit for 5 minutes to meld flavors, allowing tomatoes to release some juices.

- **Toast the Bread**: If not using freshly made *Almond-Oat Flatbread*, toast 4 slices of whole-grain bread in a toaster or oven at 350°F (175°C) for 5–7 minutes until crisp. Cut each slice in half diagonally for 8 pieces total.

- **Assemble the Bruschetta**: Spoon about 2 tablespoons of the tomato-walnut mixture onto each bread piece, pressing lightly to adhere. Arrange on a platter.

- **Serve or Store**: Serve immediately as a snack or appetizer, paired with *Pumpkin Seed Crackers* (page XX). Store leftover topping in an airtight container in the fridge for up to 2 days; assemble just before serving to prevent soggy bread.

Substitutions:

- **Cherry Tomatoes**: Diced Roma tomatoes or canned diced tomatoes (drained).

- **Walnuts**: Pecans or sunflower seeds for nut-free.

- **Balsamic Vinegar**: Red wine vinegar or lemon juice.

- **Basil**: Parsley or oregano (fresh or dried).

- **Flatbread**: Whole-grain crackers or toasted pita for convenience.

Why it Works: Tomatoes are rich in lycopene, a potent antioxidant that Dr. Li highlights in *Eat to Beat Disease* for inhibiting angiogenesis, preventing harmful blood vessel growth linked to cancer and heart disease. Walnuts provide omega-3s and ellagic acid, further supporting angiogenesis balance and heart health. Olive oil's monounsaturated fats and basil's anti-inflammatory compounds enhance cardiovascular benefits. This bruschetta is a clean, heart-healthy snack that avoids processed ingredients, aligning with Dr. Li's principles and delivering trendy walnuts in a simple, flavorful package.

Serving Suggestion: Serve with *Coconut-Cashew Yogurt* as a dip for a microbiome- and angiogenesis-boosting appetizer spread.

Grilled Salmon with Raspberry Salsa

(Dinner, angiogenesis-starving)

Prep Time: 10 minutes
Cooking Time: 15 minutes
Total Time: 25 minutes
Servings: 4 (1 fillet with ¼ cup salsa per serving)

Nutritional Information (per serving, 1 fillet with ¼ cup salsa):

- Calories: 280 kcal
- Protein: 25 g
- Fat: 16 g (2.5 g saturated)
- Carbohydrates: 8 g (3 g fiber, 3 g sugar)
- Sodium: 200 mg
- Key Nutrients: Omega-3s (30% DV), Vitamin D (20% DV), Vitamin C (15% DV) *Note*: Nutritional values are approximate, based on USDA data. Adjust for specific brands or Substitutions.

Ingredients:

- 4 salmon fillets (4–5 oz each, skin-on or skinless)
- 1 tablespoon olive oil
- ½ teaspoon salt
- ¼ teaspoon black pepper
- 1 cup fresh or frozen raspberries (thawed if frozen)
- ¼ cup red onion, finely diced
- 1 tablespoon lime juice
- 1 teaspoon fresh cilantro, chopped (or ½ teaspoon dried)
- ¼ teaspoon chili powder (optional, for heat)

Instructions:

- **Prepare the Salsa**: In a medium mixing bowl, combine raspberries, red onion, lime juice, cilantro, and chili powder (if using). Mash gently with a fork to release some juices, keeping some texture. Set aside at room temperature to meld flavors.
- **Season the Salmon**: Pat salmon fillets dry with paper towels. Brush both sides with olive oil and sprinkle with salt and pepper.
- **Grill the Salmon**: Preheat a grill pan, outdoor grill, or skillet over medium-high heat. Lightly oil the surface to prevent sticking. Place salmon fillets skin-side down (if skin-on) and cook for 4–5 minutes per side, until the flesh flakes easily with a fork and the internal temperature reaches 145°F (63°C). Avoid overcooking to keep it moist.
- **Serve**: Transfer salmon to plates and spoon ¼ cup raspberry salsa over each fillet. Serve immediately with *Spinach and Mushroom Frittata* (page XX) or steamed greens for a complete meal.

- **Store**: Store leftover salmon and salsa separately in airtight containers in the fridge for up to 2 days. Reheat salmon gently in a microwave or oven at 300°F (150°C) for 5–7 minutes; serve salsa cold or at room temperature.

Substitutions:

- **Salmon**: Trout or mackerel for similar omega-3s; tofu for plant-based (adjust cooking time).
- **Raspberries**: Strawberries or blackberries work well.
- **Red Onion**: Shallot or green onion for milder flavor.
- **Lime Juice**: Lemon juice or apple cider vinegar.
- **Cilantro**: Parsley or omit for herb-free.

Why it Works: Salmon is a Dr. Li favorite, packed with omega-3 fatty acids that inhibit angiogenesis, as noted in *Eat to Beat Disease*, starving tumors and supporting heart health. Raspberries provide ellagic acid and vitamin C, further blocking harmful blood vessel growth and protecting DNA from oxidative stress. Olive oil's monounsaturated fats and cilantro's antioxidants enhance cardiovascular benefits. This dish is a clean, angiogenesis-starving dinner that avoids processed ingredients, aligning with Dr. Li's principles and delivering a nutrient-dense, flavorful meal.

Serving Suggestion: Pair with *Brussels Sprouts with Pomegranate* for an angiogenesis- and DNA-protective dinner.

Strawberry-Arugula Salad

(Lunch, with avocado)

Prep Time: 10 minutes
Cooking Time: 0 minutes
Total Time: 10 minutes
Servings: 4 (1 cup per serving, about 4 cups total)

Nutritional Information (per serving, 1 cup):

- Calories: 160 kcal
- Protein: 3 g
- Fat: 12 g (1.5 g saturated)
- Carbohydrates: 12 g (4 g fiber, 5 g sugar)
- Sodium: 150 mg
- Key Nutrients: Vitamin C (25% DV), Vitamin K (20% DV), Folate (10% DV)

Ingredients:

- 4 cups baby arugula
- 1 cup fresh strawberries, hulled and sliced
- 1 ripe avocado, pitted, peeled, and diced
- ¼ cup walnuts, roughly chopped
- 2 tablespoons olive oil
- 1 tablespoon balsamic vinegar

- 1 teaspoon Dijon mustard
- ¼ teaspoon salt
- ⅛ teaspoon black pepper

Instructions:

- **Prepare the Salad**: In a large mixing bowl, combine arugula, sliced strawberries, diced avocado, and chopped walnuts. Toss gently to distribute ingredients evenly.
- **Make the Dressing**: In a small bowl or jar, whisk together olive oil, balsamic vinegar, Dijon mustard, salt, and black pepper until emulsified (smooth and combined). Alternatively, shake in a jar with a lid.
- **Dress the Salad**: Drizzle the dressing over the salad and toss gently to coat, being careful not to mash the avocado. Taste and adjust with more salt or vinegar if desired.
- **Serve**: Divide the salad among 4 plates or serve family-style in the mixing bowl. Enjoy immediately as a light lunch or pair with *Cottage Cheese Herb Bread* (page XX) for a heartier meal.
- **Store**: Store undressed salad components in separate airtight containers in the fridge for up to 2 days. Dress just before serving to prevent wilting. Store dressing in a jar for up to 1 week; shake before using.

Substitutions:

- **Arugula**: Baby spinach or mixed greens for a milder flavor.
- **Strawberries**: Blueberries or raspberries for similar benefits.
- **Avocado**: Sliced cucumber or Greek yogurt dollops for creaminess.
- **Walnuts**: Pecans or sunflower seeds for nut-free.
- **Balsamic Vinegar**: Lemon juice or red wine vinegar.

Why it Works: Strawberries are rich in ellagic acid and vitamin C, which Dr. Li highlights in *Eat to Beat Disease* for inhibiting angiogenesis (starving harmful blood vessels) and protecting DNA from oxidative damage. Arugula provides nitrates and folate, supporting heart health and cellular repair. Avocado and olive oil offer monounsaturated fats that promote microbiome health and vascular function, while walnuts add omega-3s for additional angiogenesis support. This salad is a clean, heart-healthy dish that avoids processed ingredients, aligning with Dr. Li's principles and delivering trendy avocado and arugula in a simple, flavorful package.

Serving Suggestion: Pair with *Pumpkin Seed Crackers* and *Coconut-Cashew Yogurt* dip for a heart- and microbiome-boosting lunch.

Green Tea Poached Chicken (Dinner, simple)

Prep Time: 10 minutes
Cooking Time: 20 minutes
Total Time: 30 minutes
Servings: 4 (1 chicken breast per serving)

Nutritional Information (per serving, 1 chicken breast):

- Calories: 180 kcal
- Protein: 26 g
- Fat: 6 g (1 g saturated)
- Carbohydrates: 2 g (0 g fiber, 1 g sugar)
- Sodium: 300 mg
- Key Nutrients: Protein (50% DV), Niacin (20% DV), Antioxidants (catechins)

Ingredients:

- 4 boneless, skinless chicken breasts (4–5 oz each)
- 4 cups water
- 2 green tea bags (or 2 tablespoons loose-leaf green tea)
- 1 tablespoon olive oil
- 1 teaspoon minced fresh ginger (or ½ teaspoon ground ginger)
- 1 garlic clove, minced
- ½ teaspoon salt
- ¼ teaspoon black pepper
- 1 tablespoon fresh parsley, chopped (optional, for garnish)

Instructions:

- **Prepare the Poaching Liquid**: In a large saucepan or deep skillet, bring 4 cups water to a simmer over medium heat (not a rolling boil). Add green tea bags (or loose-leaf tea in a strainer), ginger, garlic, and salt. Simmer for 5 minutes to infuse flavors, then remove tea bags or strainer.

- **Season the Chicken**: Pat chicken breasts dry with paper towels. Rub with olive oil and sprinkle with black pepper.

- **Poach the Chicken**: Gently place chicken breasts in the simmering tea mixture, ensuring they're fully submerged (add more water if needed). Cover and cook on low heat for 12–15 minutes, until the internal temperature reaches 165°F (74°C) and the chicken is opaque. Check doneness with a meat thermometer or by cutting into the thickest part.

- **Rest and Slice**: Remove chicken with tongs and let rest on a cutting board for 5 minutes to retain juices. Slice thinly or serve whole, garnished with parsley if desired.

- **Serve or Store**: Serve warm with *Brussels Sprouts with Pomegranate* (page XX) or shred for *Avocado-Chickpea Pita* (page XX). Store in an airtight container in the fridge for up to 3 days or freeze for up to 1 month. Reheat gently in a microwave or steamer.

Substitutions:

- **Chicken**: Turkey breast or tofu for plant-based (adjust cooking time for tofu).
- **Green Tea**: White tea or jasmine tea for similar benefits; avoid black tea (too strong).
- **Olive Oil**: Avocado oil or omit for lower fat.
- **Ginger**: Ground turmeric or omit.
- **Parsley**: Cilantro or green onion for garnish.

Why it Works: Green tea is a Dr. Li favorite, rich in catechins like EGCG that inhibit angiogenesis, as noted in *Eat to Beat Disease*, starving tumors and supporting heart health. Chicken provides lean protein for tissue repair and regeneration, while olive oil and ginger offer anti-inflammatory compounds that enhance immunity and microbiome health. This dish is a clean, angiogenesis-supporting dinner that avoids processed ingredients, aligning with Dr. Li's principles and delivering a simple, nutrient-dense meal.

Serving Suggestion: Serve with *Strawberry-Arugula Salad* for a double dose of angiogenesis and DNA protection.

Tuna-Stuffed Bell Peppers

(Lunch, omega-3s)

Prep Time: 15 minutes
Cooking Time: 0 minutes
Total Time: 15 minutes
Servings: 4 (1 stuffed pepper half per serving)

Nutritional Information (per serving, 1 stuffed pepper half):

- Calories: 200 kcal
- Protein: 15 g
- Fat: 10 g (1.5 g saturated)
- Carbohydrates: 12 g (4 g fiber, 3 g sugar)
- Sodium: 250 mg
- Key Nutrients: Omega-3s (15% DV), Vitamin C (50% DV), Protein (30% DV)

Ingredients:

- 2 large bell peppers (any color), halved and seeded
- 2 cans (5 oz each) tuna in water, drained
- 1 ripe avocado, pitted and peeled
- 1 tablespoon lemon juice
- 1 tablespoon olive oil
- ¼ cup diced celery
- 2 tablespoons chopped fresh parsley (or 1 teaspoon dried)
- ¼ teaspoon salt
- ⅛ teaspoon black pepper

- ¼ cup chopped walnuts (optional, for crunch)

Instructions:

- **Prepare the Peppers**: Slice bell peppers in half lengthwise and remove seeds and membranes. Rinse and pat dry. Arrange cut-side up on a platter or plate.
- **Make the Filling**: In a medium mixing bowl, combine drained tuna, avocado, lemon juice, olive oil, celery, parsley, salt, and black pepper. Mash with a fork or potato masher until creamy but with some texture, similar to tuna salad. Stir in walnuts, if using, for added crunch.
- **Stuff the Peppers**: Spoon about ⅓ cup of the tuna mixture into each pepper half, pressing gently to fill. Smooth the top or leave rustic.
- **Serve**: Serve immediately with *Pumpkin Seed Crackers* (page XX) or chill for up to 4 hours for a refreshing lunch. Pair with *Tomato-Walnut Bruschetta* (page XX) for a complete meal.
- **Store**: Store stuffed peppers in an airtight container in the fridge for up to 2 days. Alternatively, store filling and peppers separately for up to 3 days and assemble before serving to maintain pepper crunch.

Substitutions:

- **Bell Peppers**: Large tomatoes or cucumber boats for a different vessel.
- **Tuna**: Canned salmon or mashed chickpeas for plant-based.
- **Avocado**: Greek yogurt or hummus for creaminess.
- **Celery**: Diced cucumber or carrot for crunch.
- **Walnuts**: Sunflower seeds or omit for nut-free.

Why it Works: Tuna is a Dr. Li staple, rich in omega-3 fatty acids that inhibit angiogenesis, as noted in *Eat to Beat Disease*, supporting heart health and starving tumors. Bell peppers provide vitamin C and antioxidants for DNA protection, while avocado and olive oil offer monounsaturated fats that promote microbiome health. Walnuts (optional) add extra omega-3s and crunch. This dish is a clean, omega-3-rich lunch that avoids processed ingredients, aligning with Dr. Li's principles and delivering a nutrient-dense, no-cook meal.

Serving Suggestion: Serve with *Berry-Chia Jam* on *Almond-Oat Flatbread* for an omega-3- and DNA-protective lunch.

Cherry-Chia Pudding (Dessert, no sugar)

Prep Time: 10 minutes
Cooking Time: 0 minutes (plus 4 hours chilling)
Total Time: 10 minutes active, 4 hours total
Servings: 4 (½ cup per serving, about 2 cups total)

Nutritional Information (per serving, ½ cup):

- Calories: 130 kcal
- Protein: 4 g
- Fat: 7 g (1 g saturated)
- Carbohydrates: 14 g (5 g fiber, 6 g sugar)
- Sodium: 50 mg
- Key Nutrients: Vitamin C (10% DV), Omega-3s (8% DV), Antioxidants (anthocyanins)

Ingredients:

- 1 ½ cups frozen cherries (thawed, or fresh, pitted)
- 1 cup unsweetened almond milk
- ¼ cup chia seeds
- 1 tablespoon lemon juice
- ½ teaspoon vanilla extract
- ¼ cup chopped walnuts (optional, for topping)

Instructions:

- **Blend the Base**: In a blender or food processor, combine thawed cherries, almond milk, lemon juice, and vanilla extract. Blend on high for 30–60 seconds until smooth, with no large cherry chunks remaining.
- **Mix with Chia Seeds**: Pour the cherry mixture into a medium mixing bowl. Add chia seeds and stir well to combine. Let sit for 5 minutes, then stir again to prevent clumping.
- **Chill the Pudding**: Divide the mixture among 4 small jars or bowls. Cover and refrigerate for at least 4 hours, or overnight, until the pudding thickens to a gel-like consistency.
- **Serve**: Stir each pudding before serving to ensure even texture. Top with chopped walnuts, if using, for added crunch. Enjoy as a dessert or breakfast treat.
- **Store**: Store covered in the fridge for up to 5 days. Stir before serving, as chia seeds may settle. Not recommended for freezing, as texture may become watery.

Substitutions:

- **Cherries**: Frozen blueberries or raspberries for similar benefits.
- **Almond Milk**: Any unsweetened plant-based milk (e.g., oat, soy) or water.
- **Chia Seeds**: Ground flaxseeds can work, but texture may be less firm.

- **Lemon Juice**: Lime juice or orange juice.
- **Walnuts**: Almonds or sunflower seeds for nut-free.

Why it Works: Cherries are rich in anthocyanins and quercetin, which Dr. Li highlights in *Eat to Beat Disease* for inhibiting angiogenesis, preventing harmful blood vessel growth linked to cancer and heart disease. Chia seeds provide omega-3s and fiber, supporting microbiome health and satiety, while almond milk adds a clean, neutral base. Walnuts (optional) contribute additional omega-3s and vitamin E for DNA protection. This no-sugar pudding is a clean, angiogenesis-supporting dessert that aligns with Dr. Li's principles, delivering trendy chia seeds in a simple, nutrient-dense package.

Serving Suggestion: Pair with *Maple-Walnut Granola* for a crunchy, angiogenesis-boosting dessert or breakfast.

Roasted Tomato Soup (Lunch, with basil)

Prep Time: 10 minutes
Cooking Time: 35 minutes
Total Time: 45 minutes
Servings: 4 (1 cup per serving, about 4 cups total)

Nutritional Information (per serving, 1 cup):

- Calories: 140 kcal
- Protein: 3 g
- Fat: 8 g (1 g saturated)
- Carbohydrates: 15 g (4 g fiber, 8 g sugar)
- Sodium: 300 mg
- Key Nutrients: Lycopene (antioxidants), Vitamin C (20% DV), Vitamin A (15% DV)
  Note: Nutritional values are approximate, based on USDA data. Adjust for specific brands or Substitutions.

Ingredients:

- 2 pounds Roma tomatoes (about 8 medium), halved
- 1 small onion, quartered
- 2 garlic cloves, peeled
- 2 tablespoons olive oil
- ½ teaspoon salt
- ¼ teaspoon black pepper
- 1 cup low-sodium vegetable broth

- ¼ cup fresh basil leaves, chopped
- 1 teaspoon balsamic vinegar (optional, for depth)

Instructions:

- **Preheat Oven**: Preheat your oven to 400°F (200°C). Line a baking sheet with parchment paper or aluminum foil for easy cleanup.
- **Roast the Vegetables**: Place tomato halves, onion quarters, and garlic cloves on the baking sheet. Drizzle with 1 tablespoon olive oil and sprinkle with salt and pepper. Toss to coat, then arrange tomatoes cut-side up. Roast for 25–30 minutes, until tomatoes are soft and slightly caramelized.
- **Blend the Soup**: Transfer roasted vegetables (with juices) to a blender or medium saucepan (if using an immersion blender). Add vegetable broth and balsamic vinegar (if using). Blend until smooth, about 30–60 seconds. If using a blender, work in batches and vent the lid to avoid steam buildup.
- **Heat and Season**: Pour the blended soup into a medium saucepan (if not already there). Heat over medium-low for 5 minutes, stirring occasionally, until warmed through. Stir in chopped basil and remaining 1 tablespoon olive oil. Taste and adjust with more salt or pepper if needed.
- **Serve**: Ladle into bowls and serve with *Cottage Cheese Herb Bread* (page XX) or *Pumpkin Seed Crackers* (page XX). Garnish with extra basil if desired.
- **Store**: Store in an airtight container in the fridge for up to 4 days or freeze for up to 3 months. Reheat gently on the stovetop or microwave, stirring to combine.

Substitutions:

- **Roma Tomatoes**: Cherry tomatoes or canned whole tomatoes (reduce roasting time).
- **Onion**: Shallot or omit for milder flavor.
- **Vegetable Broth**: Water or chicken broth (if not vegetarian).
- **Basil**: Parsley or oregano (fresh or dried).
- **Olive Oil**: Avocado oil or omit for lower fat.

Why it Works: Tomatoes are a Dr. Li staple, packed with lycopene, an antioxidant that inhibits angiogenesis and protects DNA from damage, as noted in *Eat to Beat Disease*. Roasting enhances lycopene bioavailability, boosting its heart-healthy and anti-cancer effects. Basil and olive oil provide anti-inflammatory compounds and monounsaturated fats, supporting microbiome health and vascular function. This soup is a clean, angiogenesis-supporting lunch that avoids processed ingredients, aligning with Dr. Li's principles and delivering a comforting, nutrient-dense meal.

Serving Suggestion: Pair with *Strawberry-Arugula Salad* for a double dose of angiogenesis and DNA protection.

Pomegranate-Glazed Carrots (Side, vibrant)

Prep Time: 10 minutes
Cooking Time: 20 minutes
Total Time: 30 minutes
Servings: 4 (½ cup per serving, about 2 cups total)

Nutritional Information (per serving, ½ cup):

- Calories: 110 kcal
- Protein: 1 g
- Fat: 4 g (0.5 g saturated)
- Carbohydrates: 18 g (4 g fiber, 10 g sugar)
- Sodium: 200 mg
- Key Nutrients: Vitamin A (80% DV), Vitamin C (10% DV), Antioxidants (ellagic acid)

Ingredients:

- 1 pound carrots (about 4–5 medium), peeled and cut into 2-inch sticks
- 1 tablespoon olive oil
- ¼ teaspoon salt
- ⅛ teaspoon black pepper
- ¼ cup pomegranate juice (100% pure, no added sugar)
- 1 tablespoon maple syrup
- 1 teaspoon lemon juice
- 2 tablespoons pomegranate seeds (optional, for garnish)
- 1 teaspoon fresh parsley, chopped (optional, for garnish)

Instructions:

- **Preheat Oven**: Preheat your oven to 425°F (220°C). Line a baking sheet with parchment paper or aluminum foil for easy cleanup.
- **Roast the Carrots**: Place carrot sticks on the baking sheet. Drizzle with olive oil and sprinkle with salt and pepper. Toss to coat, then spread in a single layer. Roast for 15–20 minutes, flipping halfway, until tender and slightly caramelized.
- **Make the Glaze**: While carrots roast, combine pomegranate juice, maple syrup, and lemon juice in a small saucepan. Bring to a simmer over medium heat and cook for 5–7 minutes, stirring occasionally, until reduced to a thick, syrupy glaze (about 2 tablespoons).
- **Glaze the Carrots**: Remove carrots from the oven and drizzle with the pomegranate glaze. Toss to coat evenly. Return to the oven for 2–3 minutes to set the glaze.

- **Serve**: Transfer carrots to a serving dish. Garnish with pomegranate seeds and parsley, if using, for a vibrant presentation. Serve warm as a side with *Grilled Salmon with Raspberry Salsa* (page XX).
- **Store**: Store in an airtight container in the fridge for up to 4 days. Reheat in a 350°F oven for 5–7 minutes or microwave for 1–2 minutes.

Substitutions:

- **Carrots**: Parsnips or sweet potatoes (adjust roasting time).
- **Pomegranate Juice**: Cranberry juice (100% pure) or diluted red grape juice.
- **Maple Syrup**: Honey or omit for less sweetness.
- **Olive Oil**: Avocado oil or omit for lower fat.
- **Pomegranate Seeds**: Chopped dried cranberries or omit.

Why it Works: Pomegranates are rich in ellagic acid and punicalagins, which Dr. Li notes in *Eat to Beat Disease* for inhibiting angiogenesis and protecting DNA, supporting heart health and cancer prevention. Carrots provide beta-carotene and fiber, enhancing DNA protection and microbiome health. Olive oil's monounsaturated fats and parsley's antioxidants further promote vascular health. This side dish is a clean, angiogenesis-supporting addition to any meal, aligning with Dr. Li's principles and delivering trendy pomegranate in a simple, colorful package.

Serving Suggestion: Serve with *Green Tea Poached Chicken* for a vibrant, angiogenesis-focused dinner.

Blackberry-Cottage Cheese Toast (Snack)

Prep Time: 5 minutes
Cooking Time: 0 minutes
Total Time: 5 minutes
Servings: 2 (1 toast per serving)

Nutritional Information (per serving, 1 toast):

- Calories: 150 kcal
- Protein: 8 g
- Fat: 6 g (1 g saturated)
- Carbohydrates: 16 g (3 g fiber, 4 g sugar)
- Sodium: 200 mg
- Key Nutrients: Vitamin C (10% DV), Calcium (8% DV), Antioxidants (anthocyanins)

Note: Nutritional values are approximate, based on USDA data. Adjust for specific brands or Substitutions.

Ingredients:

- 2 slices *Almond-Oat Flatbread* (page XX) or whole-grain bread
- ½ cup low-fat cottage cheese

- ½ cup fresh blackberries, halved
- 1 teaspoon olive oil (optional, for drizzle)
- 1 teaspoon fresh mint, chopped (optional, for garnish)

Instructions:

- **Toast the Bread**: Toast *Almond-Oat Flatbread* or whole-grain bread in a toaster or oven at 350°F (175°C) for 5 minutes until crisp.
- **Assemble the Toast**: Spread ¼ cup cottage cheese evenly over each toast slice. Arrange blackberry halves on top, pressing gently to adhere.
- **Finish and Serve**: Drizzle with olive oil and sprinkle with mint, if using, for extra flavor and presentation. Serve immediately as a snack or light breakfast.
- **Store**: Store components separately (unassembled) in the fridge for up to 2 days. Assemble just before eating to prevent soggy bread.
- **Serving**: Cut into smaller pieces for a party appetizer.

Substitutions:

- **Blackberries**: Raspberries or blueberries for similar benefits.
- **Cottage Cheese**: Greek yogurt or *Coconut-Cashew Yogurt* (page XX) for plant-based.
- **Flatbread**: Whole-grain crackers or rye bread.
- **Olive Oil**: Omit or use a balsamic glaze drizzle.
- **Mint**: Basil or omit.

Why it Works: Blackberries are rich in anthocyanins, which Dr. Li highlights in *Eat to Beat Disease* for DNA protection and angiogenesis inhibition, supporting heart health and cancer prevention. Cottage cheese provides probiotics and protein, boosting immunity and gut health. Olive oil adds monounsaturated fats for microbiome support. This toast is a clean, immunity-boosting snack that aligns with Dr. Li's principles, delivering trendy cottage cheese in a quick, nutrient-dense package.

Serving Suggestion: Pair with *Blueberry-Spinach Smoothie* (page XX) for an immunity- and DNA-protective snack combo.

Beet Hummus (Snack, vibrant)

Prep Time: 10 minutes
Cooking Time: 0 minutes (if using pre-cooked beets)
Total Time: 10 minutes
Servings: 6 (¼ cup per serving, about 1.5 cups total)

Nutritional Information (per serving, ¼ cup):

- Calories: 120 kcal
- Protein: 4 g
- Fat: 6 g (1 g saturated)

- Carbohydrates: 14 g (4 g fiber, 3 g sugar)
- Sodium: 200 mg
- Key Nutrients: Folate (10% DV), Manganese (8% DV), Fiber (16% DV)

Ingredients:

- 1 cup canned chickpeas, rinsed and drained
- 1 medium cooked beet (about ½ cup, peeled and chopped)
- 2 tablespoons tahini
- 2 tablespoons olive oil
- 1 tablespoon lemon juice
- 1 garlic clove, minced
- ¼ teaspoon salt
- 2–3 tablespoons water (for consistency)

Instructions:

- Blend all ingredients except water in a food processor for 1–2 minutes until smooth, scraping down sides. Add water 1 tablespoon at a time, blending until creamy.
- Taste and adjust with more lemon juice or salt. Serve with *Pumpkin Seed Crackers* or veggies. Store in an airtight container in the fridge for up to 5 days.

Tips: Use pre-cooked beets (supermarket produce section) to save time. Blend longer for smoother texture. Store with a thin layer of olive oil on top to preserve freshness.

Substitutions: Swap tahini for almond butter; use roasted carrots for beets. **Why it Works**: Beets contain betalains, which Dr. Li notes support angiogenesis balance and DNA protection. Chickpeas and tahini provide fiber and prebiotics for microbiome health. This hummus is a clean, vibrant snack aligned with Dr. Li's principles.

Red Grape Sorbet (Dessert, no sugar)

Prep Time: 10 minutes
Cooking Time: 0 minutes (plus 4 hours freezing)
Total Time: 10 minutes active, 4 hours total
Servings: 4 (½ cup per serving, about 2 cups total)

Nutritional Information (per serving, ½ cup):

- Calories: 80 kcal
- Protein: 1 g
- Fat: 0 g
- Carbohydrates: 20 g (1 g fiber, 18 g sugar)
- Sodium: 0 mg
- Key Nutrients: Vitamin C (10% DV), Resveratrol (antioxidants)

Ingredients:

- 3 cups frozen red grapes

- 1 tablespoon lemon juice
- 1 teaspoon lemon zest (optional)

Instructions:

- Blend frozen grapes, lemon juice, and zest in a food processor for 1–2 minutes until smooth, scraping down sides.
- Serve immediately as soft-serve or freeze in an airtight container for 2–4 hours for firmer texture. Let soften 5 minutes before scooping. Store in the freezer for up to 1 month.

Tips: Freeze grapes ahead for instant prep. Pulse briefly to avoid over-blending. Serve in chilled bowls to maintain texture.

Substitutions: Use frozen cherries or blueberries; lime juice for lemon.

Why it Works: Red grapes are rich in resveratrol, which Dr. Li notes protects DNA and inhibits angiogenesis. This sorbet is a clean, no-sugar dessert aligned with Dr. Li's principles.

Tuna Quinoa Bowl (Lunch, omega-3s)

Prep Time: 15 minutes
Cooking Time: 0 minutes (if quinoa is pre-cooked)
Total Time: 15 minutes
Servings: 4 (1 cup per serving, about 4 cups total)

Nutritional Information (per serving, 1 cup):

- Calories: 250 kcal
- Protein: 18 g
- Fat: 10 g (1.5 g saturated)
- Carbohydrates: 22 g (5 g fiber, 2 g sugar)
- Sodium: 300 mg
- Key Nutrients: Omega-3s (15% DV), Protein (36% DV)

Ingredients:

- 1 can (5 oz) tuna in water, drained
- 2 cups cooked quinoa
- 1 avocado, diced
- 1 cup chopped cucumber
- 2 tablespoons olive oil
- 1 tablespoon lemon juice

- ¼ teaspoon salt
- 2 tablespoons fresh dill, chopped

Instructions:

- In a large bowl, combine tuna, quinoa, avocado, cucumber, olive oil, lemon juice, salt, and dill. Toss gently.
- Serve immediately or chill for up to 4 hours. Store in the fridge for up to 2 days.

Tips: Use pre-cooked quinoa for speed. Add avocado last to prevent browning.

Substitutions: Swap tuna for chickpeas; spinach for cucumber.

Why it Works: Tuna provides omega-3s for angiogenesis inhibition, while quinoa and avocado support microbiome health. This bowl is a clean, nutrient-dense lunch aligned with Dr. Li's principles.

Kale-Avocado Breakfast Bowl (Breakfast, regeneration)

Prep Time: 5 minutes
Cooking Time: 10 minutes
Total Time: 15 minutes
Servings: 2 (1 bowl per serving)

Nutritional Information (per serving):

- Calories: 280 kcal
- Protein: 12 g
- Fat: 20 g (3 g saturated)
- Carbohydrates: 15 g (6 g fiber, 2 g sugar)
- Sodium: 250 mg
- Key Nutrients: Vitamin K (50% DV), Protein (24% DV)

Ingredients:

- 2 cups chopped kale
- 1 avocado, sliced
- 2 large eggs
- 1 tablespoon olive oil
- ¼ teaspoon salt
- ⅛ teaspoon black pepper
- 1 tablespoon sunflower seeds

Instructions:

- Sauté kale in olive oil over medium heat for 3–4 minutes until wilted. Season with salt and pepper.
- Fry eggs in the same pan to desired doneness (2–3 minutes for sunny-side up).
- Divide kale and avocado between two bowls, top with eggs and sunflower seeds. Serve immediately.

Tips: Massage kale with oil for tenderness. Use pre-washed kale for speed.

Substitutions: Swap eggs for tofu; spinach for kale.

Why it Works: Kale and avocado provide nutrients for stem cell activity, supporting regeneration. Eggs add protein for tissue repair. This bowl aligns with Dr. Li's clean-eating principles.

Shiitake and Spinach Soup (Dinner, immunity)

Prep Time: 5 minutes
Cooking Time: 15 minutes
Total Time: 20 minutes
Servings: 4 (1 cup per serving)

Nutritional Information (per serving):

- Calories: 100 kcal
- Protein: 4 g
- Fat: 4 g (0.5 g saturated)
- Carbohydrates: 12 g (3 g fiber, 2 g sugar)
- Sodium: 300 mg
- Key Nutrients: Vitamin D (10% DV), Vitamin K (20% DV)

Ingredients:

- 2 cups sliced shiitake mushrooms
- 2 cups baby spinach
- 4 cups low-sodium vegetable broth
- 1 tablespoon olive oil
- 1 garlic clove, minced
- 1 teaspoon grated ginger
- ¼ teaspoon salt

Instructions:

- Sauté garlic, ginger, and mushrooms in olive oil in a saucepan over medium heat for 5 minutes.
- Add broth and salt; simmer for 10 minutes. Stir in spinach until wilted (1 minute).
- Serve hot. Store in the fridge for up to 3 days.

Tips: Use fresh shiitakes for best flavor. Add a splash of lemon juice for brightness.

Substitutions: Swap spinach for kale; button mushrooms for shiitake.

Why it Works: Shiitake mushrooms boost immunity with beta-glucans, while spinach supports DNA protection. This soup is a clean, immunity-focused meal aligned with Dr. Li's principles.

Turmeric-Ginger Roasted Cauliflower Steaks (Dinner, DNA protection)

Prep Time: 10 minutes
Cooking Time: 20 minutes
Total Time: 30 minutes
Servings: 4 (1 steak per serving)

Nutritional Information (per serving):

- Calories: 140 kcal
- Protein: 4 g
- Fat: 8 g (1 g saturated)
- Carbohydrates: 12 g (4 g fiber, 4 g sugar)
- Sodium: 200 mg
- Key Nutrients: Vitamin C (50% DV), Antioxidants (curcumin)

Ingredients:

- 1 large cauliflower head, cut into 4 (1-inch) steaks
- 2 tablespoons olive oil
- 1 teaspoon ground turmeric
- 1 teaspoon grated ginger
- ¼ teaspoon salt
- ⅛ teaspoon black pepper
- 1 tablespoon chopped parsley

Instructions:

- Preheat oven to 425°F. Toss cauliflower with olive oil, turmeric, ginger, salt, and pepper on a parchment-lined baking sheet.

- Roast for 20 minutes, flipping halfway, until golden. Garnish with parsley.

- Serve hot. Store in the fridge for up to 4 days.

Tips: Keep steaks intact by slicing carefully. Use fresh ginger for bold flavor.

Substitutions: Swap cauliflower for zucchini; ground ginger for fresh.

Why it Works: Turmeric's curcumin protects DNA, while cauliflower supports angiogenesis inhibition. This dish is a clean, vibrant dinner aligned with Dr. Li's principles.

Garlic-Herb Roasted Chickpeas
(Snack, microbiome)

Prep Time: 5 minutes
Cooking Time: 25 minutes
Total Time: 30 minutes
Servings: 4 (¼ cup per serving)

Nutritional Information (per serving):

- Calories: 130 kcal
- Protein: 5 g
- Fat: 5 g (0.5 g saturated)
- Carbohydrates: 16 g (4 g fiber, 1 g sugar)
- Sodium: 200 mg
- Key Nutrients: Fiber (16% DV), Iron (8% DV)

Ingredients:

- 1 can (15 oz) chickpeas, rinsed and drained
- 1 tablespoon olive oil
- 1 teaspoon garlic powder
- 1 teaspoon dried rosemary
- ¼ teaspoon salt

Instructions:

- Preheat oven to 400°F. Pat chickpeas dry and toss with olive oil, garlic powder, rosemary, and salt on a baking sheet.

- Roast for 25 minutes, shaking halfway, until crispy. Cool completely.

- Store in an airtight container for up to 1 week.

Tips: Dry chickpeas thoroughly for maximum crunch. Adjust spices to taste.

Substitutions: Swap rosemary for thyme; paprika for garlic powder.

Why it Works: Chickpeas provide prebiotic fiber for microbiome health, while garlic supports immunity. This snack is a clean, nutrient-dense option aligned with Dr. Li's principles.

Oyster Mushroom Tacos (Dinner, gut-friendly)

Prep Time: 10 minutes
Cooking Time: 10 minutes
Total Time: 20 minutes
Servings: 4 (2 tacos per serving)

Nutritional Information (per serving):

- Calories: 220 kcal
- Protein: 8 g
- Fat: 10 g (1 g saturated)
- Carbohydrates: 28 g (6 g fiber, 2 g sugar)
- Sodium: 300 mg
- Key Nutrients: Fiber (24% DV), Vitamin D (10% DV)

Ingredients:

- 2 cups sliced oyster mushrooms
- 4 *Chickpea Flour Tortillas* (page XX)
- 1 avocado, sliced
- 1 tablespoon olive oil
- 1 teaspoon smoked paprika
- ¼ teaspoon salt

- ½ cup shredded cabbage
- 2 tablespoons lime juice

Instructions:

- Sauté mushrooms in olive oil with paprika and salt for 5–7 minutes until golden.
- Warm tortillas in a skillet. Fill with mushrooms, avocado, cabbage, and a drizzle of lime juice.
- Serve immediately. Store components separately in the fridge for up to 3 days.

Tips: Slice mushrooms evenly for consistent cooking. Warm tortillas for flexibility.

Substitutions: Swap oyster mushrooms for portobello; lettuce for cabbage.

Why it Works: Oyster mushrooms provide beta-glucans for microbiome health, while avocado supports heart health. This taco is a clean, gut-friendly dinner aligned with Dr. Li's principles.

Berry-Coconut Popsicles (Dessert, DNA protection)

Prep Time: 10 minutes
Cooking Time: 0 minutes (plus 4 hours freezing)
Total Time: 10 minutes active, 4 hours total
Servings: 6 (1 popsicle per serving)

Nutritional Information (per serving):

- Calories: 90 kcal
- Protein: 1 g
- Fat: 6 g (4 g saturated)
- Carbohydrates: 8 g (2 g fiber, 5 g sugar)
- Sodium: 10 mg
- Key Nutrients: Vitamin C (15% DV), Antioxidants

Ingredients:

- 1 cup mixed berries (fresh or frozen)
- 1 cup full-fat coconut milk
- 1 tablespoon lemon juice
- 1 teaspoon vanilla extract

Instructions:

- Blend berries, coconut milk, lemon juice, and vanilla until smooth.
- Pour into popsicle molds and freeze for 4 hours.
- Run molds under warm water to release. Store in the freezer for up to 1 month.

Tips: Use silicone molds for easy release. Blend thoroughly for smooth texture.

Substitutions: Swap berries for mango; almond milk for coconut milk (less creamy).

Why it Works: Berries provide DNA-protective anthocyanins, while coconut milk supports microbiome health. This popsicle is a clean, kid-friendly dessert aligned with Dr. Li's principles.

Banana-Oat Muffins (Breakfast, microbiome)

Prep Time: 10 minutes
Cooking Time: 20 minutes
Total Time: 30 minutes
Servings: 12 (1 muffin per serving)

Nutritional Information (per serving):

- Calories: 140 kcal
- Protein: 4 g
- Fat: 6 g (1 g saturated)
- Carbohydrates: 20 g (3 g fiber, 6 g sugar)
- Sodium: 150 mg
- Key Nutrients: Fiber (12% DV), Potassium (8% DV)

Ingredients:

- 2 ripe bananas, mashed
- 1 cup rolled oats
- ½ cup almond flour
- 2 large eggs
- ¼ cup olive oil
- 1 teaspoon baking powder
- ½ teaspoon cinnamon
- ¼ teaspoon salt

Instructions:

- Preheat oven to 350°F. Mix all ingredients in a bowl until smooth.
- Divide batter among 12 lined muffin cups. Bake for 18–20 minutes until golden.
- Cool and store in the fridge for up to 5 days or freeze for 1 month.

Tips: Use very ripe bananas for sweetness. Don't overmix batter.

Substitutions: Swap eggs for flax eggs; oat flour for almond flour.

Why it Works: Bananas and oats provide prebiotic fiber for microbiome health, while almond flour supports DNA protection.

These muffins are a clean, nutrient-dense breakfast aligned with Dr. Li's principles.

Chapter 4: Regeneration Boost (Stem Cell Support)

Dark Chocolate-Oat Bites (Snack, No Sugar)

Prep Time: 10 minutes
Cooking Time: 0 minutes (chilling only)
Total Time: 40 minutes (includes chill time)
Servings: 12 bites

Nutritional Information (per serving):

- Calories: 120 kcal
- Protein: 3 g
- Fat: 7 g (3 g saturated)
- Carbohydrates: 14 g (2 g fiber, 1 g added sugar)
- Sodium: 40 mg
- Key Nutrients: Iron (8% DV), Magnesium (10% DV), Zinc (6% DV)

Ingredients:

- ¾ cup rolled oats (gluten-free if needed)
- ½ cup almond butter (unsweetened)
- ¼ cup unsweetened cocoa powder
- 2 tablespoons chia seeds
- 3 tablespoons maple syrup (or date syrup)
- 1 teaspoon vanilla extract
- Pinch of salt
- Optional: mini dark chocolate chips, shredded coconut

Instructions:

- Mix: In a medium bowl, combine oats, cocoa powder, chia seeds, and salt.

- Add Wet Ingredients: Stir in almond butter, maple syrup, and vanilla until a thick dough forms. If too dry, add 1 tablespoon water.

- Shape: Scoop 1 tablespoon of dough and roll into balls.
- Chill: Place bites on a parchment-lined plate and refrigerate for 30 minutes to firm up.

- Store: Keep in an airtight container in the fridge for up to 1 week.

Substitutions:

- Almond Butter: Peanut butter or cashew butter.
- Maple Syrup: Date syrup or honey (if not vegan).
- Cocoa Powder: Raw cacao powder for extra antioxidants.

Why it Works:
Dark chocolate and cocoa contain flavonoids that protect stem cells and promote healthy blood vessels. Oats add prebiotic fiber, and chia seeds deliver omega-3s for inflammation control. A perfect regeneration and angiogenesis snack!

Serving Suggestion: Enjoy with Green Tea Poached Chicken for a post-lunch treat.

Olive Oil Poached Cod (Dinner, Mediterranean)

Prep Time: 5 minutes
Cooking Time: 20 minutes
Total Time: 25 minutes
Servings: 2

Nutritional Information (per serving):
- Calories: 330 kcal
- Protein: 28 g
- Fat: 22 g (3 g saturated)
- Carbohydrates: 2 g (0 g fiber, 0 g added sugar)
- Sodium: 320 mg
- Key Nutrients: Omega-3s (800 mg), Vitamin D (60% DV), Selenium (70% DV)

Ingredients:
- 2 cod fillets (5–6 oz each)
- ½ cup extra-virgin olive oil
- 2 garlic cloves, sliced
- 2 sprigs fresh thyme or rosemary
- Zest of 1 lemon
- Salt and pepper, to taste
- Optional: olives or capers for garnish

Instructions:
- Prepare Oil Bath: In a small skillet or saucepan, heat olive oil over low heat with garlic and herbs until fragrant (about 2 minutes).

- Poach the Cod: Season cod fillets with salt and pepper. Gently place into the warm oil (should barely bubble). Cook for 12–15 minutes, spooning oil over the fish occasionally, until opaque and flakes easily.

- Serve: Transfer cod to plates, spoon some of the infused oil over the top, and sprinkle with lemon zest. Garnish with olives or capers if using.

Substitutions:
- Cod: Halibut, haddock, or any firm white fish.
- Herbs: Dried thyme or oregano if fresh isn't available.

Why it Works:
Poaching in olive oil preserves delicate omega-3 fats while adding antioxidant-rich polyphenols from the oil itself. This gentle cooking method supports heart health, immune function, and regeneration at the cellular level.

Serving Suggestion: Serve alongside Pomegranate-Glazed Carrots for an antioxidant-rich plate.

Sweet Potato and Kale Hash (Lunch, Hearty)

Prep Time: 10 minutes
Cooking Time: 20 minutes
Total Time: 30 minutes
Servings: 3

Nutritional Information (per serving):

- Calories: 260 kcal
- Protein: 7 g
- Fat: 10 g (2 g saturated)
- Carbohydrates: 36 g (6 g fiber, 5 g natural sugar)
- Sodium: 270 mg
- Key Nutrients: Vitamin A (250% DV), Vitamin C (40% DV), Manganese (30% DV)

Ingredients:

- 2 medium sweet potatoes, diced small
- 3 cups kale, chopped (stems removed)
- 1 small red onion, diced
- 2 tablespoons olive oil
- 1 teaspoon smoked paprika
- ½ teaspoon garlic powder
- Salt and pepper, to taste
- Optional: fried egg or avocado on top

Instructions:

- Roast Sweet Potatoes: Preheat oven to 400°F (200°C). Toss diced sweet potatoes with 1 tablespoon olive oil, paprika, garlic powder, salt, and pepper. Spread on a baking sheet and roast for 15 minutes, stirring halfway.

- Sauté Onion and Kale: In a skillet, heat 1 tablespoon olive oil. Add red onion and cook until soft, about 5 minutes. Stir in kale and cook until wilted, about 2 minutes.

- Combine: Toss roasted sweet potatoes into the skillet and stir well to combine.

- Serve: Plate warm, topped with a fried egg or sliced avocado if desired.

Substitutions:

- Sweet Potatoes: Regular potatoes or diced butternut squash.
- Kale: Swiss chard or spinach.

Why it Works:
Sweet potatoes are loaded with carotenoids for DNA repair and immune support, while kale adds stem cell-activating sulforaphane. Together they create a hearty, antioxidant-rich meal that fuels energy and cellular regeneration.

Serving Suggestion: Perfect with a side of Sauerkraut and Apple Slaw for a gut-healing combo.

Cocoa-Banana Smoothie (Breakfast, quick)

Prep Time: 5 minutes
Total Time: 5 minutes
Servings: 2

Nutritional Information (per serving):

- Calories: 210 kcal
- Protein: 8 g
- Fat: 4 g (1 g saturated)
- Carbohydrates: 38 g (6 g fiber, 15 g natural sugars)
- Sodium: 90 mg
- Key Nutrients: Potassium (20% DV), Magnesium (15% DV), Vitamin C (10% DV)

Ingredients:

- 1 ripe banana (fresh or frozen)
- 2 tablespoons unsweetened cocoa powder
- 1 cup unsweetened almond milk (or milk of choice)
- ¼ cup plain Greek yogurt (or plant-based alternative)
- 1 tablespoon chia seeds
- 1 teaspoon vanilla extract (optional)
- 3–4 ice cubes (if using fresh banana)

Instructions:

- **Blend:** Add all ingredients to a high-speed blender. Blend until smooth and creamy, about 30–45 seconds.
- **Adjust:** Taste and adjust sweetness if needed (add 1 teaspoon maple syrup if desired). If too thick, blend in a splash more almond milk.
- **Serve:** Pour into two glasses and serve immediately.

Substitutions:

- Banana: Swap with frozen mango or berries for a twist.
- Cocoa Powder: Cacao powder works too, adding extra antioxidants.
- Greek Yogurt: Use coconut yogurt for a dairy-free option.

Why it Works:
This smoothie balances quick-digesting carbs (banana) with protein and fiber (chia seeds and yogurt) for sustained energy. Cocoa powder adds flavonoids that boost circulation and cognitive function, aligning with food-as-medicine principles.

Serving Suggestion: Top with a sprinkle of cacao nibs or hemp seeds for extra texture and nutrients.

Spinach and Mushroom Frittata

(Breakfast, cottage cheese base)
Prep Time: 10 minutes
Cooking Time: 20 minutes
Total Time: 30 minutes
Servings: 4

Nutritional Information (per serving):
- Calories: 230 kcal
- Protein: 18 g
- Fat: 14 g (5 g saturated)
- Carbohydrates: 6 g (2 g fiber, 2 g natural sugars)
- Sodium: 320 mg
- Key Nutrients: Calcium (20% DV), Vitamin D (15% DV), Iron (10% DV)

Ingredients:
- 6 large eggs
- ½ cup cottage cheese (full-fat or 2%)
- 1 tablespoon olive oil
- 2 cups fresh spinach (roughly chopped)
- 1 cup cremini mushrooms (sliced)
- ½ teaspoon salt
- ¼ teaspoon black pepper
- ¼ teaspoon nutmeg (optional)

Instructions:

- **Prep Oven:** Preheat oven to 375°F (190°C). Grease a 9-inch pie dish or oven-safe skillet.
- **Sauté Vegetables:** Heat olive oil in a skillet over medium heat. Add mushrooms and cook until softened, about 5 minutes. Add spinach and cook until wilted, another 2 minutes. Remove from heat.
- **Make Egg Mixture:** In a bowl, whisk eggs, cottage cheese, salt, pepper, and nutmeg.
- **Assemble:** Stir sautéed vegetables into the egg mixture and pour into the prepared dish.
- **Bake:** Bake for 18–22 minutes until set and lightly golden. Let cool slightly before slicing.

Substitutions:

- Cottage Cheese: Ricotta or Greek yogurt can substitute.
- Spinach: Swap with kale or arugula.
- Mushrooms: Use zucchini or bell peppers instead.

Why it Works:
Cottage cheese packs extra protein and creaminess without needing cream. Spinach and mushrooms bring antioxidants and prebiotic fiber, fueling gut health and brain function.

Serving Suggestion: Serve with a side of mixed greens tossed in lemon vinaigrette.

Fig and Almond Tart (Dessert, whole-grain crust)

Prep Time: 20 minutes
Cooking Time: 30 minutes
Total Time: 50 minutes
Servings: 8

Nutritional Information (per serving):

- Calories: 260 kcal
- Protein: 5 g
- Fat: 15 g (5 g saturated)
- Carbohydrates: 28 g (4 g fiber, 12 g natural sugars)
- Sodium: 120 mg
- Key Nutrients: Fiber (15% DV), Vitamin E (20% DV), Calcium (8% DV)

Ingredients:

Crust:
- 1 cup almond flour
- ½ cup whole wheat pastry flour
- ¼ cup coconut oil or butter (melted)
- 2 tablespoons maple syrup
- ¼ teaspoon salt

Filling:
- ½ cup almond butter
- 2 tablespoons honey or maple syrup
- 1 tablespoon lemon juice
- 6–8 fresh figs (sliced)

Instructions:

- **Make Crust:** Preheat oven to 350°F (175°C). In a bowl, combine almond flour, whole wheat pastry flour, salt, melted coconut oil, and maple syrup. Mix until dough forms. Press evenly into a 9-inch tart pan.
- **Bake Crust:** Bake for 10–12 minutes until lightly golden. Let cool.
- **Prepare Filling:** In a small bowl, stir almond butter, honey, and lemon juice until smooth. Spread evenly over cooled crust.
- **Top:** Arrange fig slices over the almond butter filling.
- **Chill:** Refrigerate 15–20 minutes before slicing.

Substitutions:

- Almond Butter: Peanut butter or sunflower seed butter works.
- Figs: Try with fresh berries or thinly sliced pears.
- Coconut Oil: Avocado oil can substitute.

Why it Works:
Almonds provide vitamin E and healthy fats that promote skin health and support angiogenesis balance. Figs add natural sweetness, fiber, and prebiotics for a happy gut.

Serving Suggestion: Dust with a little cinnamon or drizzle with extra honey before serving.

Lentil-Pumpkin Stew (Dinner, cozy)

Prep Time: 15 minutes
Cooking Time: 35 minutes
Total Time: 50 minutes
Servings: 6

Nutritional Information (per serving):

- Calories: 290 kcal
- Protein: 16 g
- Fat: 6 g (1 g saturated)
- Carbohydrates: 40 g (11 g fiber, 4 g natural sugars)
- Sodium: 360 mg
- Key Nutrients: Iron (25% DV), Vitamin A (90% DV), Folate (35% DV)

Ingredients:

- 1 tablespoon olive oil
- 1 medium onion (chopped)
- 3 cloves garlic (minced)
- 1 cup brown or green lentils (rinsed)
- 2 cups diced pumpkin (or butternut squash)
- 1 teaspoon ground cumin
- ½ teaspoon smoked paprika
- 4 cups vegetable broth
- 1 cup water
- 2 cups chopped kale or spinach
- Salt and pepper, to taste

Instructions:

- **Sauté Base:** In a large pot, heat olive oil over medium heat. Add onion and garlic; cook until fragrant, about 5 minutes.
- **Add Lentils and Spices:** Stir in lentils, cumin, and smoked paprika; cook for 1 minute.
- **Simmer:** Add broth, water, and diced pumpkin. Bring to a boil, then reduce heat and simmer, covered, for 30 minutes until lentils and pumpkin are tender.
- **Finish:** Stir in kale or spinach and cook for another 5 minutes until wilted. Season with salt and pepper.

Substitutions:

- Lentils: Swap with canned beans for faster prep (reduce broth slightly).
- Pumpkin: Use sweet potato or carrots if out of season.
- Kale: Spinach or Swiss chard works too.

Why it Works:
Lentils are loaded with fiber, iron, and plant protein, perfect for gut health and energy. Pumpkin brings beta-carotene to boost immunity and vision, while the spices add anti-inflammatory power.

Serving Suggestion: Top with a dollop of plain yogurt or a squeeze of fresh lemon for brightness.

Apple-Walnut Salad

(Lunch, regeneration-focused)
Prep Time: 10 minutes
Total Time: 10 minutes
Servings: 2

Nutritional Information (per serving):

- Calories: 280 kcal
- Protein: 5 g
- Fat: 18 g (2 g saturated)
- Carbohydrates: 28 g (5 g fiber, 18 g natural sugars)
- Sodium: 120 mg
- Key Nutrients: Vitamin C (20% DV), Omega-3s (from walnuts, 10% DV), Fiber (20% DV)

Ingredients:

- 2 medium apples (crisp varieties like Honeycrisp or Gala), thinly sliced
- ½ cup walnut halves (toasted)
- 4 cups mixed greens (arugula, spinach, or mesclun)
- ¼ cup crumbled feta or goat cheese (optional)
- 2 tablespoons extra-virgin olive oil
- 1 tablespoon apple cider vinegar
- 1 teaspoon Dijon mustard
- 1 teaspoon maple syrup
- Salt and pepper, to taste

Instructions:

- **Make Dressing:** In a small jar, shake together olive oil, apple cider vinegar, Dijon mustard, maple syrup, salt, and pepper until emulsified.
- **Assemble Salad:** In a large bowl, toss greens, apple slices, walnuts, and cheese (if using).
- **Dress:** Drizzle with dressing and toss gently to coat. Serve immediately.

Substitutions:

- Walnuts: Swap with pecans or pumpkin seeds for a nut-free version.
- Apple: Pears or persimmons are delicious seasonal swaps.
- Greens: Use shredded cabbage or kale for a heartier salad.

Why it Works:
Apples are rich in polyphenols supporting regeneration at the cellular level. Walnuts offer omega-3s critical for brain and tissue health. This salad is light but nutrient-dense, making it perfect for recovery days.

Serving Suggestion: Sprinkle with a handful of pomegranate seeds for an extra burst of antioxidants.

Roasted Parsnips with Thyme

(Side, comfort food)
Prep Time: 10 minutes
Cooking Time: 25 minutes
Total Time: 35 minutes
Servings: 4

Nutritional Information (per serving):

- Calories: 160 kcal
- Protein: 2 g
- Fat: 7 g (1 g saturated)
- Carbohydrates: 24 g (6 g fiber, 5 g natural sugars)
- Sodium: 180 mg
- Key Nutrients: Fiber (20% DV), Vitamin C (15% DV), Manganese (10% DV)

Ingredients:

- 1 pound parsnips, peeled and cut into sticks
- 1 tablespoon olive oil
- 1 teaspoon fresh thyme leaves (or ½ teaspoon dried thyme)
- ½ teaspoon salt
- ¼ teaspoon pepper

Instructions:

- **Preheat Oven:** 400°F (200°C).
- **Toss Parsnips:** In a large bowl, toss parsnip sticks with olive oil, thyme, salt, and pepper.
- **Roast:** Spread in a single layer on a baking sheet. Roast for 20–25 minutes, flipping halfway, until golden and tender.

Substitutions:
- Parsnips: Use carrots, sweet potatoes, or turnips.
- Thyme: Try rosemary, sage, or a sprinkle of smoked paprika instead.

Why it Works:
Parsnips are a fantastic source of fiber and antioxidants that support digestion and immunity. Roasting brings out their natural sweetness, making them cozy and satisfying.

Serving Suggestion: Serve alongside roasted chicken, lentil loaf, or a hearty grain bowl.

Almond Butter Cups

(Dessert)
Prep Time: 15 minutes
Chill Time: 30 minutes
Total Time: 45 minutes
Servings: 12 mini cups

Nutritional Information (per mini cup):

- Calories: 120 kcal
- Protein: 3 g
- Fat: 9 g (2.5 g saturated)
- Carbohydrates: 6 g (1 g fiber, 4 g natural sugars)
- Sodium: 20 mg
- Key Nutrients: Magnesium (10% DV), Vitamin E (8% DV)

Ingredients:

- ¾ cup almond butter (unsweetened)

- 2 tablespoons maple syrup
- 1 tablespoon coconut flour (optional, for thickening)
- 1 cup dark chocolate chips (70% cocoa or higher)
- 1 tablespoon coconut oil

Instructions:

- **Make Filling:** In a bowl, mix almond butter, maple syrup, and coconut flour until smooth.
- **Melt Chocolate:** In a double boiler or microwave, melt chocolate chips with coconut oil until glossy.
- **Assemble Cups:** Spoon a little melted chocolate into the bottom of mini muffin liners. Freeze for 5 minutes to set. Add a small dollop of almond butter mixture, then cover with more melted chocolate.
- **Chill:** Freeze for 30 minutes until firm. Store in the fridge.

Substitutions:

- Almond Butter: Peanut, cashew, or sunflower seed butter works.
- Chocolate Chips: Use sugar-free chocolate if needed.

Why it Works:
Almonds bring healthy fats and magnesium to help regulate mood, muscle function, and blood sugar. These cups satisfy cravings without the crash.

Serving Suggestion: Sprinkle with flaky sea salt before the chocolate sets for extra flavor pop.

Kale Chips

(Snack, crunchy and light)

Prep Time: 10 minutes
Cooking Time: 15 minutes
Total Time: 25 minutes
Servings: 4

Nutritional Information (per serving):

- Calories: 90 kcal
- Protein: 4 g
- Fat: 4 g (0.5 g saturated)
- Carbohydrates: 8 g (2 g fiber, 1 g natural sugars)
- Sodium: 180 mg
- Key Nutrients: Vitamin K (over 100% DV), Vitamin A (80% DV), Iron (10% DV)

Ingredients:

- 1 bunch curly kale, stems removed and torn into bite-sized pieces
- 1 tablespoon olive oil
- ½ teaspoon sea salt
- ¼ teaspoon garlic powder (optional)

Instructions:

- **Preheat Oven:** 300°F (150°C).
- **Massage Kale:** Toss kale with olive oil, salt, and garlic powder. Massage gently with your hands for about 1 minute.
- **Bake:** Spread on a parchment-lined baking

sheet in a single layer. Bake for 12–15 minutes, flipping once, until crispy but not burned.

Substitutions:
- Kale: Try collard greens or Swiss chard leaves.
- Seasoning: Sprinkle with nutritional yeast for a "cheesy" flavor.

Why it Works:
Kale is a nutrient powerhouse rich in antioxidants and anti-inflammatory compounds, supporting joint, heart, and skin health.

Serving Suggestion: Enjoy immediately or store in an airtight container for up to 2 days.

Golden Turmeric Quinoa

(Side or Light Lunch, anti-inflammatory)

Prep Time: 5 minutes
Cooking Time: 15 minutes
Total Time: 20 minutes
Servings: 4

Nutritional Information (per serving):
- Calories: 210 kcal
- Protein: 7 g
- Fat: 6 g (1 g saturated)
- Carbohydrates: 30 g (3 g fiber)
- Sodium: 170 mg
- Key Nutrients: Iron (15% DV), Magnesium (20% DV), Fiber (12% DV)

Ingredients:
- 1 cup quinoa (rinsed)
- 2 cups vegetable broth (or water)
- 1 tablespoon olive oil
- 1 teaspoon turmeric powder
- ½ teaspoon cumin
- ¼ teaspoon black pepper
- ¼ teaspoon sea salt
- 2 tablespoons chopped fresh parsley or cilantro
- Optional garnish: lemon wedges

Instructions:
- **Cook Quinoa:** Bring quinoa and broth to a boil. Reduce heat to low, cover, and simmer for 15 minutes until water is absorbed.
- **Season:** Fluff quinoa with a fork. Stir in olive oil, turmeric, cumin, black pepper, and sea salt while still warm.
- **Finish:** Fold in fresh herbs. Serve warm or at room temperature with lemon wedges.

Substitutions:
- **Quinoa:** Millet or couscous can be used for a softer texture, though quinoa offers higher protein.
- **Olive Oil:** Avocado oil or flaxseed oil works for a different flavor.
- **Vegetable Broth:** Use plain water if broth isn't available, but adjust salt to taste.
- **Fresh Herbs:** Swap parsley/cilantro with mint, basil, or dill for a twist.

Serving Suggestions:

• Serve alongside grilled vegetables or roasted salmon for a balanced meal.
• Stuff into bell peppers and bake for a quinoa-stuffed veggie lunch.
• Add to leafy greens with chickpeas for a hearty salad bowl.

Why it Works:

Turmeric's curcumin compounds fight inflammation and oxidative stress, while quinoa delivers complete protein, fiber, and important minerals like magnesium. Black pepper enhances turmeric absorption. Together, they create a nutrient-dense, anti-inflammatory powerhouse.

Zucchini Ribbon Salad with Lemon-Pepper Dressing

(Fresh Side, light & hydrating)

Prep Time: 10 minutes
Total Time: 10 minutes
Servings: 2

Nutritional Information (per serving):

• Calories: 90 kcal
• Protein: 2 g
• Fat: 7 g (1 g saturated)
• Carbohydrates: 6 g (2 g fiber)
• Sodium: 150 mg
• Key Nutrients: Vitamin C (25% DV), Potassium (10% DV)

Ingredients:

• 2 medium zucchinis
• 2 tablespoons extra-virgin olive oil
• 1 tablespoon fresh lemon juice
• ½ teaspoon cracked black pepper
• ¼ teaspoon sea salt
• 1 tablespoon pine nuts or chopped almonds (optional)

Instructions:

• **Prep Zucchini:** Use a vegetable peeler to shave zucchini into long, thin ribbons.
• **Make Dressing:** Whisk olive oil, lemon juice, black pepper, and salt in a small bowl.
• **Assemble:** Toss zucchini ribbons gently with the dressing. Sprinkle with nuts if desired. Serve immediately.

Substitutions:

• **Zucchini:** Try cucumber ribbons for a similar crisp texture.
• **Olive Oil:** Walnut oil or avocado oil for a nutty twist.
• **Pine Nuts:** Substitute with pumpkin seeds or sunflower seeds for nut-free options.
• **Lemon Juice:** Lime juice adds a slightly different brightness.

Serving Suggestions:

• Pair with grilled chicken or tofu for a light lunch.
• Serve on a platter topped with feta crumbles for a fresh party appetizer.

- Mix with cooked quinoa for a heartier, protein-packed salad.

Why it Works:

Zucchini is rich in water and fiber for hydration and digestion, while lemon and black pepper bring antioxidants and gentle detox support. Olive oil adds healthy monounsaturated fats for brain and heart health.

Sweet Potato and Black Bean Tacos

(Dinner or Lunch, hearty and grounding)

Prep Time: 10 minutes
Cooking Time: 25 minutes
Total Time: 35 minutes
Servings: 4 (2 tacos per serving)

Nutritional Information (per serving):

- Calories: 320 kcal
- Protein: 11 g
- Fat: 8 g (1.5 g saturated)
- Carbohydrates: 48 g (9 g fiber)
- Sodium: 250 mg
- Key Nutrients: Fiber (30% DV), Vitamin A (300% DV), Iron (15% DV)

Ingredients:

- 2 medium sweet potatoes, peeled and diced small
- 1 tablespoon olive oil
- 1 teaspoon smoked paprika
- 1 teaspoon ground cumin
- ½ teaspoon sea salt
- 1 (15 oz) can black beans, drained and rinsed
- 8 small corn tortillas
- Optional toppings: sliced avocado, fresh salsa, chopped cilantro

Instructions:

- **Roast Sweet Potatoes:** Preheat oven to 400°F (200°C). Toss diced sweet potatoes with olive oil, paprika, cumin, and salt. Spread evenly on a baking sheet and roast 20–25 minutes until tender and lightly crispy.
- **Heat Black Beans:** Warm beans in a small saucepan over low heat.
- **Assemble Tacos:** Layer roasted sweet potatoes and black beans into warmed tortillas. Add desired toppings.

Substitutions:

- **Sweet Potatoes:** Use butternut squash cubes or roasted carrots for variation.
- **Corn Tortillas:** Flour tortillas or grain-free almond tortillas work if needed.
- **Black Beans:** Pinto beans or chickpeas make good substitutes.

- **Spices:** Add chili powder or cayenne for extra heat.

Serving Suggestions:

- Serve with a side of guacamole or cashew sour cream.
- Add shredded cabbage or pickled onions for crunch and tang.
- Turn leftovers into a taco salad over greens with lime vinaigrette.

Why it Works:

Sweet potatoes are packed with beta-carotene and slow-digesting carbs for lasting energy, while black beans provide gut-friendly fiber and plant protein. Together, they form a deeply nourishing and satisfying plant-based meal.

Chapter 5: Hearty and Healthy Comfort Foods

Wild Mushroom Stir Fry

(Vibrant, nutrient-dense, gut-healthy)

Prep Time: 10 minutes
Cooking Time: 15 minutes
Total Time: 25 minutes
Servings: 2

Nutritional Information (per serving):

- Calories: 280 kcal
- Protein: 10 g
- Fat: 18 g (2 g saturated)
- Carbohydrates: 22 g (5 g fiber, 6 g sugars)
- Sodium: 420 mg
- Key Nutrients: Vitamin D (35% DV), Potassium (18% DV), Antioxidants (from mushrooms)

Ingredients:

- 2 cups mixed wild mushrooms (shiitake, oyster, maitake, or any preferred mix), cleaned and sliced
- 1 tablespoon sesame oil (or olive oil)
- 2 cloves garlic, minced
- 1/4 cup yellow onion, thinly sliced
- 1 tablespoon soy sauce (or tamari for gluten-free)
- 1 teaspoon rice vinegar
- 1/2 teaspoon grated fresh ginger
- 1 tablespoon sesame seeds (optional, for garnish)
- Fresh cilantro (optional, for garnish)

Instructions:

1. **Prepare the Ingredients:**
   Clean and slice the mushrooms into bite-sized pieces. Mince the garlic and slice the onion. Grate the fresh ginger.

2. **Heat the Pan:**
   In a large skillet or wok, heat sesame oil over medium-high heat. Once hot, add the garlic and onion. Stir-fry for about 2 minutes until the onions begin to soften.

3. **Cook the Mushrooms:**
   Add the mushrooms to the pan, stirring well to coat them in the oil. Cook for 6–8 minutes until the mushrooms release their moisture and begin to brown slightly.

4. **Add Flavorings:**
   Stir in the soy sauce, rice vinegar, and fresh ginger. Cook for an additional 2–3 minutes, allowing the flavors to meld together and the liquid to reduce slightly.

5. **Finish and Garnish:**
   Remove from heat and garnish with sesame seeds and fresh cilantro, if desired.

6. **Serve:**
   Serve this stir fry on its own, or pair with

brown rice or quinoa for added fiber and protein. Enjoy hot!

Substitutions:

- **Mushrooms:** If wild mushrooms aren't available, you can substitute with cremini, button, or portobello mushrooms.
- **Sesame Oil:** You can use olive oil or avocado oil instead of sesame oil, though it won't have quite the same depth of flavor.
- **Soy Sauce:** For a soy-free version, use coconut aminos, which has a similar flavor profile but is gluten- and soy-free.

Serving Suggestions:

- Serve over a bed of steamed brown rice or quinoa for added nutrition.
- Pair with a side of miso soup or a simple green salad for a light, balanced meal.
- Add sautéed spinach or bok choy on the side for an extra veggie boost.

Why it Works:

Mushrooms, particularly wild varieties like shiitake and maitake, are not only rich in fiber but also contain beta-glucans — compounds that support immune function and gut health. The sesame oil brings heart-healthy fats, while the soy sauce provides an umami-rich base, enhancing the depth of flavor. Ginger and garlic add anti-inflammatory benefits and antioxidants, making this stir fry a nutrient-dense meal that supports digestion, immunity, and overall vitality.

Baked Sweet Potato with Tahini Drizzle

Prep Time: 5 minutes
Cooking Time: 45 minutes
Total Time: 50 minutes
Servings: 2

Nutritional Information (per serving):

- Calories: 350 kcal
- Protein: 6 g
- Fat: 18 g (3 g saturated)
- Carbohydrates: 46 g (7 g fiber, 12 g sugars)
- Sodium: 210 mg
- Key Nutrients: Vitamin A (120% DV), Potassium (15% DV), Healthy fats from tahini

Ingredients:

- 2 medium sweet potatoes, scrubbed clean
- 2 tablespoons tahini (sesame paste)
- 1 tablespoon lemon juice
- 1 teaspoon maple syrup (or honey)
- 1/4 teaspoon ground cumin (optional)
- Salt and pepper, to taste

- Fresh parsley or cilantro, chopped (for garnish)

Instructions:

1. **Preheat the Oven:**
   Preheat your oven to 400°F (200°C). Place a sheet of parchment paper or a baking mat on a baking tray.

2. **Prepare the Sweet Potatoes:**
   Using a fork, prick the sweet potatoes a few times on all sides. Place them on the prepared baking tray and bake for 40–45 minutes, until the sweet potatoes are soft and tender when pierced with a fork.

3. **Make the Tahini Drizzle:**
   While the sweet potatoes are baking, prepare the tahini drizzle. In a small bowl, whisk together tahini, lemon juice, maple syrup, and cumin. Add a little water if needed to reach a smooth, pourable consistency. Season with salt and pepper to taste.

4. **Serve:**
   Once the sweet potatoes are baked and tender, slice them open and fluff the insides with a fork. Drizzle with the tahini sauce, and garnish with freshly chopped parsley or cilantro.

5. **Enjoy:**
   Serve as a side dish, or pair with a protein like grilled chicken or chickpeas for a complete meal.

Substitutions:

- **Sweet Potatoes:** You can substitute with yams, but sweet potatoes provide a creamier texture.
- **Tahini:** If you don't have tahini, you can use almond butter or cashew butter as an alternative.
- **Maple Syrup:** Use honey or agave nectar if you prefer a different sweetener.
- **Lemon Juice:** Lime juice works just as well if you want a citrusy twist.

Serving Suggestions:

- Serve alongside grilled chicken, chickpeas, or a simple salad for a well-rounded meal.
- Top with sautéed greens (like kale or spinach) for a heartier dish.
- For a comforting bowl, serve with a dollop of Greek yogurt or a sprinkle of feta cheese.

Why it Works:

Sweet potatoes are an excellent source of beta-carotene (vitamin A), which supports immune function and skin health. The tahini drizzle adds healthy fats and a creamy texture, while lemon juice enhances the flavor profile and provides a dose of vitamin C. This dish is also rich in fiber, supporting digestion and gut health, making it a satisfying and nourishing meal. The natural sweetness of the potatoes balances perfectly with the tahini's earthy richness, creating a delicious and nutritious dish that's easy to prepare and full of flavor.

Turmeric Chicken Skillet

(Flavor-packed, anti-inflammatory, one-pan meal)

Prep Time: 10 minutes
Cooking Time: 20 minutes
Total Time: 30 minutes
Servings: 2

Nutritional Information (per serving):

- Calories: 350 kcal
- Protein: 32 g
- Fat: 20 g (5 g saturated)
- Carbohydrates: 8 g (2 g fiber, 3 g sugars)
- Sodium: 300 mg
- Key Nutrients: Vitamin C (15% DV), Iron (12% DV), Omega-3s

Ingredients:

- 2 boneless, skinless chicken breasts (about 6 oz each)
- 1 tablespoon olive oil (for cooking)
- 1 teaspoon ground turmeric
- 1 teaspoon paprika
- 1/2 teaspoon cumin
- 1/2 teaspoon garlic powder
- Salt and pepper, to taste
- 1/2 cup coconut milk (or any milk of choice)
- 1 tablespoon fresh lemon juice
- Fresh cilantro, chopped (for garnish)
- Optional: 1 tablespoon chopped almonds (for crunch)

Instructions:

1. **Prepare the Chicken:** Season the chicken breasts on both sides with turmeric, paprika, cumin, garlic powder, salt, and pepper.

2. **Heat the Skillet:** In a large skillet, heat the olive oil over medium-high heat. Once hot, add the seasoned chicken breasts and cook for 6-7 minutes per side until they are golden brown and fully cooked through (internal temperature should reach 165°F). Remove the chicken from the skillet and set it aside.

3. **Make the Sauce:** In the same skillet, pour in the coconut milk and scrape up any flavorful bits stuck to the pan. Stir in the lemon juice and cook for 2-3 minutes, allowing the sauce to reduce slightly and thicken.

4. **Combine:**
Return the cooked chicken breasts to the skillet, spooning some of the sauce over them. Let the chicken simmer in the sauce for another 2 minutes to absorb the flavors.

5. **Serve:**
   Garnish with freshly chopped cilantro and optional almonds for added texture. Serve immediately.

Substitutions:

- **Chicken Breasts:** Skinless chicken thighs work well in this recipe, offering a slightly juicier texture.

- **Olive Oil:** You can substitute with avocado oil or coconut oil for cooking.

- **Coconut Milk:** Use dairy milk or any plant-based milk if you prefer a different base for the sauce.

- **Turmeric:** If you don't have ground turmeric, you can use curry powder, though the flavor will be slightly different.

Serving Suggestions:

- Serve this dish over a bed of cauliflower rice or quinoa to make it a more filling meal.

- Pair with a side of sautéed greens like spinach or kale for added nutrients and fiber.

- Add a fresh salad with a tangy vinaigrette to balance the richness of the turmeric sauce.

Why it Works:

Turmeric is known for its powerful anti-inflammatory properties, and when combined with healthy fats from coconut milk, it creates a dish that is both flavorful and nourishing. The chicken provides lean protein, supporting muscle repair and satiety. The addition of lemon juice adds brightness, balancing the richness of the coconut milk, while the spices like cumin and paprika bring warmth and depth to the dish. This skillet meal is easy to prepare, packed with flavor, and supports overall health with its combination of anti-inflammatory ingredients.

Grilled Salmon with Broccoli Salsa

(Protein-rich, omega-3 powerhouse)

Prep Time: 10 minutes
Cooking Time: 12 minutes
Total Time: 22 minutes
Servings: 2

Nutritional Information (per serving):

- Calories: 420 kcal

- Protein: 38 g

- Fat: 24 g (5 g saturated)

- Carbohydrates: 8 g (3 g fiber, 2 g sugars)

- Sodium: 310 mg

- Key Nutrients: Omega-3 Fatty Acids (EPA/DHA), Vitamin C (45% DV), Selenium (55% DV)

Ingredients:

- 2 salmon fillets (about 5 oz each), preferably wild-caught
- 2 teaspoons olive oil
- 1/2 teaspoon sea salt
- 1/4 teaspoon black pepper
- 1 cup broccoli florets, finely chopped
- 1/4 cup red onion, finely diced
- 1 small jalapeño, seeded and finely chopped (optional for spice)
- 2 tablespoons fresh cilantro, chopped
- Juice of 1 lime
- 1 tablespoon extra-virgin olive oil (for salsa)

Instructions:

1. **Preheat the Grill:** Heat a grill pan or outdoor grill to medium-high. Brush the salmon fillets with olive oil and season with salt and pepper.
2. **Prepare Broccoli Salsa:** In a medium bowl, combine chopped broccoli, red onion, jalapeño (if using), cilantro, lime juice, and 1 tablespoon olive oil. Toss gently and season with a pinch of salt.
3. **Grill the Salmon:** Place salmon skin-side down on the grill. Cook for 4–5 minutes, until the flesh is opaque halfway up the side. Flip carefully and cook another 3–4 minutes, depending on thickness, until fully cooked but still moist.
4. **Assemble and Serve:** Plate the salmon and generously spoon the broccoli salsa over the top. Serve immediately.

Substitutions:

- **Salmon:** Swap for arctic char, steelhead trout, or even grilled tofu steaks for a plant-based version.
- **Broccoli:** Finely chopped raw cauliflower makes a good substitute.
- **Lime Juice:** Lemon juice works fine in place of lime.

Serving Suggestions:

- Serve with quinoa or brown rice for extra fiber and minerals.
- Pair with roasted sweet potatoes for a complete anti-inflammatory plate.
- Garnish with extra lime wedges and microgreens for a fresh finish.

Why it Works:

Wild salmon is loaded with bioavailable omega-3s, crucial for reducing inflammation, supporting brain health, and enhancing regenerative capacity. Broccoli, when eaten raw, offers high levels of sulforaphane — a potent phytochemical shown to activate cellular detox pathways and protect DNA. The lime juice adds vitamin C, enhancing iron absorption and boosting immune health. This quick, nutrient-dense meal aligns with food-as-medicine principles, offering delicious protection against chronic disease while fueling vibrant energy.

Lentil & Eggplant Shepherd's Pie

(Plant-based comfort food with hearty lentils and eggplant)

Prep Time: 20 minutes
Cooking Time: 40 minutes
Total Time: 1 hour
Servings: 4

Nutritional Information (per serving):

- Calories: 280 kcal
- Protein: 15 g
- Fat: 12 g (2 g saturated)
- Carbohydrates: 35 g (9 g fiber, 8 g sugars)
- Sodium: 400 mg
- Key Nutrients: Fiber (36% DV), Iron (15% DV), Vitamin A (10% DV)

Ingredients:

- 1 large eggplant, diced
- 1 cup cooked lentils (or 1 can, drained and rinsed)
- 1 onion, chopped
- 2 garlic cloves, minced
- 2 tablespoons tomato paste
- 1 tablespoon olive oil
- 1 teaspoon ground cumin
- 1 teaspoon paprika
- 1/2 teaspoon dried thyme
- 1/2 cup vegetable broth
- 1/2 cup unsweetened almond milk (or any milk of choice)
- 1/4 cup nutritional yeast (optional, for a cheesy flavor)
- Salt and pepper to taste
- 2 large potatoes, peeled and boiled until soft
- 2 tablespoons vegan butter or olive oil (for mashed potatoes)

Instructions:

1. **Prepare the Eggplant:** Heat 1 tablespoon of olive oil in a large skillet over medium heat. Add the diced eggplant and cook for 8-10 minutes until tender and golden brown. Set aside.

2. **Cook the Lentil Filling:** In the same skillet, sauté the onion and garlic until soft, about 5 minutes. Add the tomato paste, cumin, paprika, and thyme, and cook for 1-2 minutes. Add the cooked lentils and vegetable broth. Stir and simmer for 5-7 minutes to combine the flavors. Season with salt and pepper.

3. **Mash the Potatoes:** Mash the boiled potatoes with the almond milk and vegan butter until smooth. Add salt and pepper to taste. You can also stir in nutritional yeast for a cheesy flavor.

4. **Assemble the Shepherd's Pie:** Preheat the oven to 375°F (190°C). In a baking dish, layer the lentil mixture first, then top with the sautéed eggplant. Spread the mashed potatoes evenly on top.

5. **Bake:**
Place the assembled shepherd's pie in the oven and bake for 20-25 minutes until the top is golden and crispy. Let it cool for a few minutes before serving.

Substitutions:

- **Eggplant:** Zucchini can be used as a substitute if eggplant is not available.
- **Vegan Butter:** Any plant-based butter or olive oil can replace the vegan butter in the mashed potatoes.
- **Lentils:** You can substitute lentils with chickpeas or black beans for a different texture.

Serving Suggestions:

- Serve with a side of sautéed greens like spinach or kale for extra nutrients.
- Pair with a fresh salad or a tangy dressing to balance the richness of the pie.

Why it Works:

This plant-based shepherd's pie is a perfect comfort food option, packed with fiber from lentils and eggplant. The creamy mashed potatoes provide a satisfying topping, while the spices like cumin and paprika infuse the dish with warm flavors. Nutritional yeast gives it a cheesy depth without any dairy, and the hearty lentils provide plant-based protein, making this a nutritious and filling meal.

Cauliflower Steaks with Pesto

(A light yet satisfying vegetarian entrée)

Prep Time: 10 minutes
Cooking Time: 20 minutes
Total Time: 30 minutes
Servings: 2

Nutritional Information (per serving):

- Calories: 250 kcal
- Protein: 8 g
- Fat: 20 g (3 g saturated)
- Carbohydrates: 12 g (5 g fiber, 5 g sugars)
- Sodium: 300 mg
- Key Nutrients: Vitamin C (80% DV), Vitamin K (15% DV), Fiber (20% DV)

Ingredients:

- 1 medium cauliflower, cut into 1-inch steaks
- 2 tablespoons olive oil

- Salt and pepper to taste
- 1/4 cup fresh basil leaves
- 2 tablespoons pine nuts (or walnuts)
- 1 garlic clove
- 2 tablespoons nutritional yeast (optional, for a cheesy flavor)
- 2 tablespoons olive oil (for pesto)
- 1 tablespoon lemon juice

Instructions:

1. **Prepare the Cauliflower Steaks:** Preheat the oven to 400°F (200°C). Cut the cauliflower into 1-inch thick steaks, trying to keep them intact. Brush both sides with olive oil and season with salt and pepper.

2. **Roast the Cauliflower:** Place the cauliflower steaks on a baking sheet and roast for 20-25 minutes, flipping halfway, until golden brown and tender.

3. **Make the Pesto:** In a food processor, combine basil, pine nuts, garlic, nutritional yeast, olive oil, and lemon juice. Pulse until smooth. Add a pinch of salt and pepper to taste.

4. **Serve:** Top each cauliflower steak with a generous spoonful of pesto and serve warm.

Substitutions:

- **Pine Nuts:** Walnuts or almonds can be used as alternatives to pine nuts in the pesto.
- **Nutritional Yeast:** If you prefer a dairy-based version, Parmesan cheese can be substituted.
- **Cauliflower:** Broccoli or zucchini steaks can be used if you prefer.

Serving Suggestions:

- Serve the cauliflower steaks with a side of quinoa or couscous to make the meal more substantial.
- Pair with a side salad dressed with a tangy lemon vinaigrette for a refreshing contrast.

Why it Works:

Cauliflower is a nutrient-dense, low-calorie vegetable that roasts beautifully, becoming caramelized and full of flavor. The pesto adds a creamy, herby element to the dish, rich in healthy fats from olive oil and pine nuts. This dish is perfect for anyone looking for a low-carb, plant-based option with plenty of healthy fats and antioxidants.

Black Garlic Roasted Chicken

(Rich in flavor with a savory depth from black garlic)

Prep Time: 10 minutes
Cooking Time: 45 minutes
Total Time: 55 minutes
Servings: 4

Nutritional Information (per serving):

- Calories: 380 kcal
- Protein: 30 g
- Fat: 25 g (5 g saturated)
- Carbohydrates: 8 g (2 g fiber, 4 g sugars)
- Sodium: 400 mg
- Key Nutrients: Protein (60% DV), Iron (12% DV), Vitamin B6 (20% DV)

Ingredients:

- 4 chicken thighs (bone-in, skin-on)
- 3 tablespoons black garlic paste (or 6 cloves black garlic, mashed)
- 1 tablespoon olive oil
- 1 teaspoon lemon zest
- 1 teaspoon fresh thyme leaves
- 1 teaspoon smoked paprika
- Salt and pepper to taste

Instructions:

1. **Prepare the Chicken:** Preheat the oven to 400°F (200°C). Pat the chicken thighs dry with paper towels. In a small bowl, combine black garlic paste, olive oil, lemon zest, thyme, paprika, salt, and pepper. Rub this mixture all over the chicken thighs.

2. **Roast the Chicken:** Place the chicken thighs on a baking sheet and roast for 35-40 minutes, or until the skin is crispy and the chicken is fully cooked (internal temperature should reach 165°F).

3. **Serve:** Let the chicken rest for a few minutes before serving. Garnish with additional thyme and lemon slices if desired.

Substitutions:

- **Chicken Thighs:** Bone-in, skinless chicken thighs or chicken breasts can be used.
- **Black Garlic:** If you can't find black garlic, you can use regular garlic, though the flavor will be less complex.

Serving Suggestions:

- Pair with roasted vegetables like carrots or Brussels sprouts for a balanced, nutrient-packed meal.

- Serve with a side of mashed cauliflower or a whole grain like quinoa for a complete dinner.

Why it Works:

Black garlic adds a sweet, umami-rich flavor that elevates the chicken, providing deep complexity without being overpowering. The healthy fats from olive oil and the protein from chicken thighs make this a satisfying meal. The roasted skin gets crispy, while the meat remains juicy and tender, perfect for a delicious, comforting dish.

Bok Choy & Tofu Stir Fry

(A quick, plant-based meal packed with vitamins)

Prep Time: 10 minutes
Cooking Time: 10 minutes
Total Time: 20 minutes
Servings: 2

Nutritional Information (per serving):

- Calories: 250 kcal
- Protein: 16 g
- Fat: 18 g (3 g saturated)
- Carbohydrates: 10 g (4 g fiber, 5 g sugars)
- Sodium: 350 mg
- Key Nutrients: Calcium (20% DV), Vitamin A (50% DV), Fiber (15% DV)

Ingredients:

- 1 block firm tofu, drained and cubed
- 1 tablespoon sesame oil
- 2 cups bok choy, chopped
- 1 tablespoon soy sauce (or tamari for gluten-free)
- 1 tablespoon rice vinegar
- 1 teaspoon sesame seeds (for garnish)
- 1 teaspoon grated ginger
- 2 garlic cloves, minced

Instructions:

1. **Prepare the Tofu:**
   In a non-stick skillet, heat sesame oil over medium-high heat. Add the cubed tofu and cook until golden brown on all sides, about 5-7 minutes. Remove and set aside.

2. **Stir Fry the Vegetables:**
   In the same skillet, add a bit more sesame oil if needed and sauté garlic and ginger for 1 minute until fragrant. Add the bok choy and cook for 3-4 minutes until wilted but still vibrant green.

3. **Combine:**
   Add the tofu back into the skillet and pour in the soy sauce and rice vinegar. Toss everything together and cook for another 2-3 minutes.

4. **Serve:**
   Garnish with sesame seeds and serve immediately.

Substitutions:

- **Tofu:** Tempeh or edamame can replace tofu for a different texture.
- **Bok Choy:** Use spinach, kale, or any leafy green as a substitute for bok choy.

Serving Suggestions:

- Serve over brown rice or quinoa for a filling, balanced meal.
- Pair with a miso soup or Asian-style salad for a complete meal.

Why it Works:

This stir fry is full of plant-based protein from tofu, combined with bok choy's rich vitamins and minerals. Sesame oil adds healthy fats and depth of flavor, while the soy sauce and rice vinegar balance the dish with umami and acidity. It's a quick and nutritious option for a busy weeknight.

Chapter 6: DNA Defense (Anti-Cancer and Anti-Aging)

Turmeric-Ginger Oatmeal

(Breakfast, anti-inflammatory)

Prep Time: 5 minutes
Cooking Time: 10 minutes
Total Time: 15 minutes
Servings: 2 (1 cup per serving, about 2 cups total)

Nutritional Information (per serving, 1 cup):

- Calories: 200 kcal
- Protein: 6 g
- Fat: 6 g (1 g saturated)
- Carbohydrates: 32 g (5 g fiber, 6 g sugar)
- Sodium: 150 mg
- Key Nutrients: Fiber (20% DV), Manganese (15% DV), Antioxidants (curcumin)

Ingredients:

- 1 cup rolled oats (gluten-free if needed)
- 2 cups unsweetened almond milk (or water)
- 1 teaspoon ground turmeric
- 1 teaspoon grated fresh ginger (or ½ teaspoon ground ginger)
- 1 tablespoon maple syrup (optional, for sweetness)
- ¼ teaspoon ground cinnamon
- ¼ teaspoon salt
- 2 tablespoons chopped walnuts (optional, for topping)

Instructions:

- **Cook the Oats**: In a small saucepan, combine almond milk, rolled oats, turmeric, ginger, cinnamon, and salt. Bring to a gentle simmer over medium heat, stirring occasionally to prevent sticking.
- **Simmer and Stir**: Reduce heat to low and cook for 8–10 minutes, stirring frequently, until the oats are tender and the mixture is creamy. If too thick, add 1–2 tablespoons more almond milk or water.
- **Sweeten and Serve**: Remove from heat and stir in maple syrup, if using. Divide between two bowls and top with walnuts, if desired, for added crunch. Serve warm.
- **Store**: Store leftovers in an airtight container in the fridge for up to 3 days. Reheat on the stovetop or microwave with a splash of milk to revive creaminess.

Substitutions:

- **Rolled Oats**: Steel-cut oats (increase cooking time to 20 minutes) or quick oats (reduce to 5 minutes).

- **Almond Milk**: Any unsweetened plant-based milk (e.g., oat, soy) or water.
- **Maple Syrup**: Omit or use honey (not vegan) or a mashed banana.
- **Walnuts**: Pumpkin seeds or almonds for nut-free.
- **Turmeric/Ginger**: Use ½ teaspoon curry powder for a different anti-inflammatory profile.

Why it Works: Turmeric's curcumin and ginger's gingerol are potent anti-inflammatory compounds that Dr. Li highlights in *Eat to Beat Disease* for protecting DNA and reducing chronic inflammation linked to disease. Oats provide prebiotic fiber to support microbiome health, while walnuts (optional) add omega-3s for angiogenesis balance. This oatmeal is a clean, anti-inflammatory breakfast that avoids processed ingredients, aligning with Dr. Li's principles and delivering trendy turmeric in a simple, nutrient-dense dish.

Serving Suggestion: Pair with *Blueberry-Spinach Smoothie* for an anti-inflammatory and DNA-protective breakfast combo.

Broccoli-Avocado Salad

(Lunch, with lemon)

Prep Time: 10 minutes
Cooking Time: 5 minutes
Total Time: 15 minutes
Servings: 4 (1 cup per serving, about 4 cups total)

Nutritional Information (per serving, 1 cup):

- Calories: 180 kcal
- Protein: 4 g
- Fat: 14 g (2 g saturated)
- Carbohydrates: 12 g (5 g fiber, 2 g sugar)
- Sodium: 200 mg
- Key Nutrients: Vitamin C (50% DV), Vitamin K (30% DV), Fiber (20% DV) *Note*: Nutritional values are approximate, based on USDA data. Adjust for specific brands or Substitutions.

Ingredients:

- 4 cups broccoli florets (fresh or frozen, thawed)
- 1 ripe avocado, pitted, peeled, and diced
- ¼ cup sunflower seeds
- 2 tablespoons olive oil
- 2 tablespoons lemon juice
- 1 teaspoon Dijon mustard
- ¼ teaspoon salt

- ⅛ teaspoon black pepper

Instructions:

- **Cook the Broccoli**: Bring a medium saucepan of water to a boil or set up a steamer. Add broccoli florets and blanch or steam for 3–4 minutes until bright green and crisp-tender. Drain and rinse under cold water to stop cooking. Pat dry.

- **Prepare the Salad**: In a large mixing bowl, combine broccoli, diced avocado, and sunflower seeds. Toss gently to distribute.

- **Make the Dressing**: In a small bowl or jar, whisk together olive oil, lemon juice, Dijon mustard, salt, and black pepper until emulsified. Alternatively, shake in a jar with a lid.

- **Dress and Serve**: Drizzle the dressing over the salad and toss gently to coat, being careful not to mash the avocado. Serve immediately or chill for up to 1 hour for enhanced flavor.

- **Store**: Store undressed salad components in separate airtight containers in the fridge for up to 3 days. Dress just before serving to maintain texture. Store dressing in a jar for up to 1 week; shake before using.

Substitutions:

- **Broccoli**: Cauliflower or green beans for similar crunch.

- **Avocado**: Mashed Greek yogurt or hummus for creaminess.

- **Sunflower Seeds**: Pumpkin seeds or chopped almonds.

- **Lemon Juice**: Lime juice or apple cider vinegar.

- **Olive Oil**: Avocado oil or omit for lower fat.

Why it Works: Broccoli is rich in sulforaphane, which Dr. Li notes in *Eat to Beat Disease* for inhibiting angiogenesis and protecting DNA, supporting cancer prevention and heart health. Avocado provides monounsaturated fats and fiber for microbiome health, while sunflower seeds add vitamin E for immunity. Lemon juice enhances nutrient absorption and adds antioxidants. This salad is a clean, heart-healthy lunch that avoids processed ingredients, aligning with Dr. Li's principles and delivering trendy avocado in a nutrient-dense package.

Serving Suggestion: Pair with *Cottage Cheese Herb Bread* for a heart- and immunity-boosting lunch.

Grilled Mackerel with Citrus

(Dinner, omega-3s)

Prep Time: 10 minutes
Cooking Time: 10 minutes
Total Time: 20 minutes
Servings: 4 (1 fillet per serving)

Nutritional Information (per serving, 1 fillet):

- Calories: 250 kcal
- Protein: 22 g
- Fat: 16 g (3 g saturated)
- Carbohydrates: 4 g (1 g fiber, 2 g sugar)
- Sodium: 200 mg
- Key Nutrients: Omega-3s (30% DV), Vitamin D (15% DV), Vitamin C (10% DV)
  Note: Nutritional values are approximate, based on USDA data. Adjust for specific brands or Substitutions.

Ingredients:

- 4 mackerel fillets (4–5 oz each, skin-on)
- 1 tablespoon olive oil
- ½ teaspoon salt
- ¼ teaspoon black pepper
- 1 orange, zested and juiced (about ¼ cup juice)
- 1 tablespoon lemon juice
- 1 teaspoon fresh thyme, chopped (or ½ teaspoon dried)
- 1 tablespoon chopped parsley (optional, for garnish)

Instructions:

- **Prepare the Citrus Topping**: In a small bowl, whisk together orange juice, orange zest, lemon juice, and thyme. Set aside to meld flavors.
- **Season the Mackerel**: Pat mackerel fillets dry with paper towels. Brush both sides with olive oil and sprinkle with salt and pepper.
- **Grill the Mackerel**: Preheat a grill pan, outdoor grill, or skillet over medium-high heat. Lightly oil the surface to prevent sticking. Place fillets skin-side down and cook for 4–5 minutes per side, until the flesh flakes easily with a fork and the internal temperature reaches 145°F (63°C). Avoid overcooking to keep it moist.
- **Serve**: Transfer fillets to plates and spoon 1–2 tablespoons of the citrus topping over each. Garnish with parsley, if using. Serve immediately with *Pomegranate-Glazed Carrots* (page XX) for a complete meal.
- **Store**: Store leftover mackerel and citrus topping separately in airtight containers in the fridge for up to 2 days. Reheat mackerel gently in a microwave or oven

at 300°F (150°C) for 5 minutes; serve topping cold or at room temperature.

Substitutions:

- **Mackerel**: Sardines or salmon for similar omega-3s; tofu for plant-based (adjust cooking time).
- **Orange Juice**: Grapefruit or lime juice for a different citrus note.
- **Thyme**: Rosemary or oregano (fresh or dried).
- **Olive Oil**: Avocado oil or omit for lower fat.
- **Parsley**: Cilantro or omit.

Why it Works: Mackerel is a Dr. Li favorite, packed with omega-3 fatty acids that inhibit angiogenesis, as noted in *Eat to Beat Disease*, starving tumors and supporting heart health. Citrus juice provides vitamin C and flavonoids for DNA protection, while olive oil and thyme offer anti-inflammatory compounds for microbiome health. This dish is a clean, omega-3-rich dinner that avoids processed ingredients, aligning with Dr. Li's principles and delivering a nutrient-dense, flavorful meal.

Serving Suggestion: Serve with *Strawberry-Arugula Salad* for an omega-3- and angiogenesis-supporting dinner.

Cauliflower Steaks with Tahini

(Dinner, with peanut butter substitute)

Prep Time: 10 minutes
Cooking Time: 20 minutes
Total Time: 30 minutes
Servings: 4 (1 steak per serving)

Nutritional Information (per serving, 1 steak):

- Calories: 200 kcal
- Protein: 6 g
- Fat: 14 g (2 g saturated)
- Carbohydrates: 14 g (5 g fiber, 4 g sugar)
- Sodium: 250 mg
- Key Nutrients: Vitamin C (60% DV), Fiber (20% DV), Vitamin E (10% DV)

Ingredients:

- 1 large cauliflower head, cut into 4 (1-inch) steaks
- 2 tablespoons olive oil
- ½ teaspoon smoked paprika
- ¼ teaspoon salt
- ⅛ teaspoon black pepper

- 2 tablespoons almond butter (substitute for tahini)
- 1 tablespoon lemon juice
- 2–3 tablespoons water (for sauce consistency)
- 1 tablespoon chopped parsley (optional, for garnish)

Instructions:

- **Preheat Oven**: Preheat your oven to 425°F (220°C). Line a baking sheet with parchment paper or aluminum foil for easy cleanup.
- **Prepare Cauliflower Steaks**: Trim leaves and stem from cauliflower, keeping the core intact. Slice into 4 (1-inch) steaks; some florets may break off (roast these alongside). Place steaks on the baking sheet, drizzle with 1 tablespoon olive oil, and sprinkle with smoked paprika, salt, and pepper. Rub to coat evenly.
- **Roast the Steaks**: Roast for 20–25 minutes, flipping halfway, until golden brown and tender. Check doneness with a fork; edges should be slightly crisp.
- **Make the Almond Butter Sauce**: In a small bowl, whisk together almond butter, lemon juice, remaining 1 tablespoon olive oil, and 2 tablespoons water until smooth. Add more water, 1 teaspoon at a time, for a drizzleable consistency. Taste and adjust with more lemon juice or salt if needed.
- **Serve**: Place cauliflower steaks on plates and drizzle with almond butter sauce. Garnish with parsley, if using. Serve warm with *Tuna Quinoa Bowl* (page XX) for a complete meal.
- **Store**: Store leftover steaks and sauce separately in airtight containers in the fridge for up to 4 days. Reheat steaks in a 350°F oven for 5–7 minutes; serve sauce cold or at room temperature.

Substitutions:

- **Cauliflower**: Zucchini or portobello mushrooms (adjust roasting time).
- **Almond Butter**: Cashew butter or sunflower seed butter for nut-free; tahini if preferred.
- **Lemon Juice**: Lime juice or apple cider vinegar.
- **Olive Oil**: Avocado oil or omit for lower fat.
- **Smoked Paprika**: Chili powder or turmeric for different flavor profiles.

Why it Works: Cauliflower is rich in sulforaphane, which Dr. Li notes in *Eat to Beat Disease* for inhibiting angiogenesis and protecting DNA, supporting cancer prevention and heart health. Almond butter provides healthy fats and vitamin E for immunity and microbiome health, while lemon juice enhances nutrient absorption with antioxidants. Smoked paprika adds anti-inflammatory compounds. This dish is a clean, angiogenesis-supporting dinner that avoids processed ingredients, aligning with

Dr. Li's principles and delivering a trendy plant-based option.

Serving Suggestion: Pair with *Cherry-Chia Pudding* for a DNA-protective dinner and dessert combo.

Cinnamon-Roasted Pears

(Dessert, no sugar)

Prep Time: 10 minutes
Cooking Time: 20 minutes
Total Time: 30 minutes
Servings: 4 (1 pear half per serving)

Nutritional Information (per serving, 1 pear half):

- Calories: 100 kcal
- Protein: 1 g
- Fat: 4 g (0.5 g saturated)
- Carbohydrates: 17 g (4 g fiber, 10 g sugar)
- Sodium: 50 mg
- Key Nutrients: Fiber (16% DV), Vitamin C (10% DV), Antioxidants (polyphenols)

Ingredients:

- 2 ripe but firm pears (e.g., Bosc or Anjou), halved and cored
- 1 tablespoon olive oil
- 1 teaspoon ground cinnamon
- ¼ teaspoon salt
- 2 tablespoons chopped pecans (optional, for topping)
- 1 teaspoon fresh rosemary, chopped (optional, for garnish)

Instructions:

- **Preheat Oven**: Preheat your oven to 375°F (190°C). Line a baking sheet with parchment paper or aluminum foil for easy cleanup.
- **Prepare the Pears**: Place pear halves cut-side up on the baking sheet. Drizzle with olive oil and sprinkle with cinnamon and salt. Rub gently to coat evenly.
- **Roast the Pears**: Roast for 20–25 minutes, until pears are tender and slightly caramelized. Check doneness with a fork; they should be soft but hold their shape.
- **Serve**: Transfer pear halves to plates and top with pecans and rosemary, if using, for added texture and flavor. Serve warm as a dessert or breakfast topping.
- **Store**: Store in an airtight container in the fridge for up to 4 days. Reheat in a 350°F oven for 5 minutes or serve cold.

Substitutions:

- **Pears**: Apples or peaches (adjust roasting time slightly).
- **Olive Oil**: Avocado oil or omit for lower fat.
- **Cinnamon**: Cardamom or allspice for a different warm spice.

- **Pecans**: Walnuts or sunflower seeds for nut-free.
- **Rosemary**: Mint or omit.

Why it Works: Pears are rich in fiber and polyphenols, which Dr. Li notes in *Eat to Beat Disease* for supporting microbiome health and inhibiting angiogenesis, promoting heart health and cancer prevention. Cinnamon provides anti-inflammatory compounds, while pecans (optional) add healthy fats and vitamin E for DNA protection. Olive oil enhances nutrient absorption. This dessert is a clean, no-sugar treat that aligns with Dr. Li's principles, delivering a simple, nutrient-dense indulgence.

Serving Suggestion: Serve with *Cocoa-Hazelnut Spread* for a microbiome- and regeneration-friendly dessert.

Brussels Sprouts with Pomegranate

(Side, festive)

Prep Time: 10 minutes
Cooking Time: 20 minutes
Total Time: 30 minutes
Servings: 4 (¾ cup per serving, about 3 cups total)

Nutritional Information (per serving, ¾ cup):

- Calories: 140 kcal
- Protein: 4 g
- Fat: 8 g (1 g saturated)
- Carbohydrates: 16 g (5 g fiber, 6 g sugar)
- Sodium: 200 mg
- Key Nutrients: Vitamin C (60% DV), Vitamin K (50% DV), Antioxidants (ellagic acid)

Ingredients:

- 1 pound Brussels sprouts, trimmed and halved
- ½ cup pomegranate seeds (from 1 small pomegranate or pre-seeded pack)
- 2 tablespoons olive oil
- ½ teaspoon salt
- ¼ teaspoon black pepper
- 1 tablespoon balsamic vinegar
- 2 tablespoons chopped walnuts (optional, for crunch)

Instructions:

- **Preheat Oven**: Preheat your oven to 425°F (220°C). Line a baking sheet with parchment paper or aluminum foil for easy cleanup.
- **Prepare Brussels Sprouts**: In a large mixing bowl, toss Brussels sprouts with olive oil, salt, and black pepper until evenly coated. Spread in a single layer on the baking sheet, cut-side down for maximum caramelization.
- **Roast**: Roast for 20–25 minutes, flipping halfway, until golden brown and crispy on the edges. Check doneness with a

fork; they should be tender but not mushy.

- **Add Pomegranate and Finish**: Transfer roasted Brussels sprouts back to the mixing bowl. Add pomegranate seeds, balsamic vinegar, and walnuts (if using). Toss gently to combine.

- **Serve**: Serve warm or at room temperature as a festive side with *Grilled Salmon with Raspberry Salsa* (page XX). Garnish with extra pomegranate seeds for presentation, if desired.

- **Store**: Store in an airtight container in the fridge for up to 4 days. Reheat in a 350°F oven for 5–7 minutes or serve cold as a salad.

Substitutions:

- **Brussels Sprouts**: Broccoli florets or cauliflower (adjust roasting time).
- **Pomegranate Seeds**: Dried cranberries or chopped red grapes.
- **Olive Oil**: Avocado oil or omit for lower fat.
- **Balsamic Vinegar**: Lemon juice or apple cider vinegar.
- **Walnuts**: Pecans or sunflower seeds for nut-free.

Why it Works: Brussels sprouts are rich in glucosinolates, which Dr. Li highlights in *Eat to Beat Disease* for inhibiting angiogenesis and supporting DNA protection, aiding cancer prevention and heart health. Pomegranate seeds provide ellagic acid and punicalagins for additional angiogenesis inhibition and antioxidant support. Olive oil and walnuts (optional) offer monounsaturated fats and omega-3s for microbiome health. This festive side is a clean, nutrient-dense dish that aligns with Dr. Li's principles, delivering trendy pomegranate in a vibrant, flavorful package.

Serving Suggestion: Pair with *Green Tea Poached Chicken* for a festive, angiogenesis-focused meal.

Chickpea Patties with Spinach

(Lunch)

Prep Time: 10 minutes
Cooking Time: 15 minutes
Total Time: 25 minutes
Servings: 4 (2 patties per serving, 8 patties total)

Nutritional Information (per serving, 2 patties):

- Calories: 220 kcal
- Protein: 9 g
- Fat: 10 g (1.5 g saturated)
- Carbohydrates: 25 g (7 g fiber, 2 g sugar)
- Sodium: 300 mg
- Key Nutrients: Fiber (28% DV), Iron (15% DV), Vitamin K (20% DV)

Ingredients:

- 1 can (15 oz) chickpeas, rinsed and drained
- 1 cup fresh baby spinach, chopped
- ½ cup rolled oats (gluten-free if needed)
- 1 small onion, finely diced
- 1 garlic clove, minced
- 2 tablespoons olive oil (1 for patties, 1 for cooking)
- 1 teaspoon ground cumin
- ½ teaspoon salt
- ¼ teaspoon black pepper
- 1 tablespoon lemon juice

Instructions:

- **Prepare the Mixture**: In a food processor or large mixing bowl, pulse or mash chickpeas until mostly smooth with some texture. Add chopped spinach, oats, onion, garlic, 1 tablespoon olive oil, cumin, salt, pepper, and lemon juice. Pulse or mix until combined; the mixture should hold together when pressed.
- **Form Patties**: Divide the mixture into 8 equal portions and shape into patties (about 2 inches wide, ½ inch thick). If too sticky, wet your hands slightly.
- **Cook the Patties**: Heat 1 tablespoon olive oil in a large skillet over medium heat. Cook patties in batches, 3–4 minutes per side, until golden brown and crispy. Avoid overcrowding; add more oil if needed.
- **Serve**: Serve warm with *Almond-Oat Flatbread* (page XX) or atop *Strawberry-Arugula Salad* (page XX). Pair with a dollop of *Coconut-Cashew Yogurt* for creaminess.
- **Store**: Store cooked patties in an airtight container in the fridge for up to 4 days or freeze for up to 1 month. Reheat in a skillet or 350°F oven for 5–7 minutes.

Substitutions:

- **Chickpeas**: White beans or lentils (cooked).
- **Spinach**: Kale or arugula, finely chopped.
- **Rolled Oats**: Breadcrumbs or almond flour (not gluten-free).
- **Olive Oil**: Avocado oil or omit for oil-free (bake at 375°F for 20 minutes, flipping halfway).
- **Cumin**: Coriander or chili powder.

Why it Works: Chickpeas are rich in prebiotic fiber, which Dr. Li notes in *Eat to Beat Disease* for supporting microbiome health and immunity. Spinach provides vitamin K and folate for DNA protection, while oats add fiber for satiety and heart health. Olive oil and cumin offer anti-inflammatory compounds. These patties are a clean, budget-friendly lunch that aligns with Dr. Li's principles, delivering nutrient-dense, plant-based protein in a simple, versatile format.

Serving Suggestion: Serve with *Pumpkin Seed Crackers* and *Beet Hummus* for a microbiome- and immunity-boosting lunch spread.

Orange-Zest Chia Pudding

(Dessert, DNA-protective)

Prep Time: 10 minutes
Cooking Time: 0 minutes (plus 4 hours chilling)
Total Time: 10 minutes active, 4 hours total
Servings: 4 (½ cup per serving, about 2 cups total)

Nutritional Information (per serving, ½ cup):

- Calories: 120 kcal
- Protein: 4 g
- Fat: 7 g (1 g saturated)
- Carbohydrates: 12 g (5 g fiber, 4 g sugar)
- Sodium: 50 mg
- Key Nutrients: Vitamin C (15% DV), Omega-3s (8% DV), Fiber (20% DV)

Ingredients:

- 1 ½ cups unsweetened almond milk
- ¼ cup chia seeds
- 1 orange, zested and juiced (about ¼ cup juice)
- ½ teaspoon vanilla extract
- ¼ teaspoon ground cinnamon (optional, for warmth)
- 2 tablespoons sliced almonds (optional, for topping)

Instructions:

- **Mix the Pudding**: In a medium mixing bowl, whisk together almond milk, chia seeds, orange juice, orange zest, vanilla extract, and cinnamon (if using). Stir well to prevent clumping. Let sit for 5 minutes, then stir again to ensure even distribution.
- **Chill**: Divide the mixture among 4 small jars or bowls. Cover and refrigerate for at least 4 hours, or overnight, until the pudding thickens to a gel-like consistency.
- **Serve**: Stir each pudding before serving to ensure even texture. Top with sliced almonds, if using, for crunch. Enjoy chilled as a dessert or breakfast.
- **Store**: Store covered in the fridge for up to 5 days. Stir before serving, as chia seeds may settle. Not recommended for freezing, as texture may become watery.

Substitutions:

- **Almond Milk**: Any unsweetened plant-based milk (e.g., oat, soy) or water.

- **Chia Seeds**: Ground flaxseeds (texture may be less firm).
- **Orange**: Lemon or grapefruit (adjust zest and juice).
- **Almonds**: Sunflower seeds or chopped walnuts for nut-free.
- **Cinnamon**: Nutmeg or omit.

Why it Works: Oranges are rich in vitamin C and flavonoids, which Dr. Li highlights in *Eat to Beat Disease* for protecting DNA from oxidative damage and inhibiting angiogenesis, supporting heart health and cancer prevention. Chia seeds provide omega-3s and fiber for microbiome health, while almonds (optional) add vitamin E for immunity. This no-sugar pudding is a clean, DNA-protective dessert that aligns with Dr. Li's principles, delivering trendy chia seeds in a simple, nutrient-dense package.

Serving Suggestion: Pair with *Blackberry-Cottage Cheese Toast* (page XX) for a DNA- and immunity-boosting dessert and snack combo.

Cabbage and Apple Stir-Fry

(Side, crunchy)

Prep Time: 5 minutes
Cooking Time: 10 minutes
Total Time: 15 minutes
Servings: 4 (¾ cup per serving, about 3 cups total)

Nutritional Information (per serving, ¾ cup):

- Calories: 110 kcal
- Protein: 2 g
- Fat: 4 g (0.5 g saturated)
- Carbohydrates: 18 g (4 g fiber, 10 g sugar)
- Sodium: 200 mg
- Key Nutrients: Vitamin C (40% DV), Fiber (16% DV), Antioxidants (polyphenols)

Ingredients:

- 4 cups shredded green cabbage (about ½ small head)
- 1 large apple (e.g., Granny Smith or Honeycrisp), cored and thinly sliced
- 1 tablespoon olive oil
- 1 tablespoon apple cider vinegar
- ½ teaspoon salt
- ¼ teaspoon black pepper
- 1 teaspoon caraway seeds (optional, for flavor)
- 1 tablespoon chopped parsley (optional, for garnish)

Instructions:

- **Heat the Pan**: Heat olive oil in a large skillet or wok over medium-high heat until shimmering.

- **Stir-Fry Cabbage**: Add shredded cabbage and caraway seeds (if using). Stir-fry for 5–7 minutes, stirring occasionally, until cabbage softens slightly but retains crunch.
- **Add Apples**: Add sliced apples, apple cider vinegar, salt, and black pepper. Stir-fry for 2–3 minutes, until apples are warmed through but still crisp.
- **Serve**: Transfer to a serving dish and garnish with parsley, if using. Serve warm or at room temperature as a side with *Chickpea Patties with Spinach* (page XX).
- **Store**: Store in an airtight container in the fridge for up to 3 days. Reheat in a skillet over medium heat for 2–3 minutes or serve cold as a slaw.

Substitutions:

- **Cabbage**: Red cabbage or kale (adjust cooking time).
- **Apple**: Pear or jicama for similar crunch.
- **Olive Oil**: Avocado oil or omit for oil-free (use a splash of water to sauté).
- **Apple Cider Vinegar**: Lemon juice or white wine vinegar.
- **Caraway Seeds**: Fennel seeds or omit.

Why it Works: Cabbage is rich in fiber and glucosinolates, which Dr. Li notes in *Eat to Beat Disease* for supporting microbiome health and DNA protection, aiding digestion and cancer prevention. Apples provide polyphenols and vitamin C for additional DNA protection and heart health. Olive oil enhances nutrient absorption with monounsaturated fats. This stir-fry is a clean, crunchy side that aligns with Dr. Li's principles, delivering a nutrient-dense, budget-friendly dish.

Serving Suggestion: Serve with *Grilled Mackerel with Citrus* (page XX) for a microbiome- and omega-3-rich meal.

Turmeric Tea Latte

(Drink, soothing)

Prep Time: 5 minutes
Cooking Time: 5 minutes
Total Time: 10 minutes
Servings: 2 (1 cup per serving, about 2 cups total)

Nutritional Information (per serving, 1 cup):

- Calories: 80 kcal
- Protein: 2 g
- Fat: 4 g (1 g saturated)
- Carbohydrates: 10 g (1 g fiber, 6 g sugar)
- Sodium: 100 mg
- Key Nutrients: Vitamin C (5% DV), Antioxidants (curcumin), Manganese (8% DV)

Ingredients:

- 2 cups unsweetened almond milk
- 1 teaspoon ground turmeric

- ½ teaspoon ground cinnamon
- ½ teaspoon grated fresh ginger (or ¼ teaspoon ground ginger)
- 1 tablespoon maple syrup (optional, for sweetness)
- ⅛ teaspoon black pepper (enhances turmeric absorption)
- ½ teaspoon vanilla extract (optional, for depth)

Instructions:

- **Heat the Milk**: In a small saucepan, combine almond milk, turmeric, cinnamon, ginger, black pepper, and vanilla extract (if using). Heat over medium-low, stirring occasionally, until steaming but not boiling, about 4–5 minutes.
- **Sweeten and Blend**: Remove from heat and stir in maple syrup, if using. For a smoother texture, blend the mixture in a blender for 20–30 seconds or use an immersion blender. If using fresh ginger, strain through a fine mesh strainer to remove pulp, if desired.
- **Serve**: Pour into two mugs and serve warm. Sprinkle with a pinch of cinnamon for garnish, if desired.
- **Store**: Store leftovers in an airtight container in the fridge for up to 3 days. Reheat gently on the stovetop or microwave, stirring to combine.

Substitutions:

- **Almond Milk**: Any unsweetened plant-based milk (e.g., oat, soy) or water.
- **Maple Syrup**: Honey (not vegan) or omit for no sweetness.
- **Turmeric**: ½ teaspoon curry powder for a different anti-inflammatory profile.
- **Ginger**: Ground allspice or omit.
- **Cinnamon**: Nutmeg or omit.

Why it Works: Turmeric's curcumin is a potent anti-inflammatory compound that Dr. Li highlights in *Eat to Beat Disease* for protecting DNA and reducing chronic inflammation linked to disease. Black pepper enhances curcumin absorption, while ginger and cinnamon add additional anti-inflammatory and antioxidant benefits. Almond milk provides a clean, neutral base for microbiome health.

Serving Suggestion: Pair with *Banana-Oat Muffins* (page XX) for an anti-inflammatory breakfast or snack.

Roasted Radishes with Garlic (Side, vibrant)

Prep Time: 5 minutes
Cooking Time: 20 minutes
Total Time: 25 minutes
Servings: 4 (½ cup per serving, about 2 cups total)

Nutritional Information (per serving, ½ cup):

- Calories: 90 kcal
- Protein: 1 g
- Fat: 7 g (1 g saturated)
- Carbohydrates: 6 g (2 g fiber, 2 g sugar)
- Sodium: 200 mg
- Key Nutrients: Vitamin C (15% DV), Antioxidants (glucosinolates)

Ingredients:

- 1 pound radishes, trimmed and halved
- 2 garlic cloves, minced
- 2 tablespoons olive oil
- ½ teaspoon salt
- ¼ teaspoon black pepper
- 1 teaspoon fresh rosemary, chopped (or ½ teaspoon dried)
- 1 tablespoon lemon juice (optional, for brightness)

Instructions:

- Preheat oven to 425°F (220°C). Line a baking sheet with parchment paper.
- Toss radishes with olive oil, garlic, salt, pepper, and rosemary on the baking sheet. Spread in a single layer.
- Roast for 20–25 minutes, stirring halfway, until tender and slightly caramelized.
- Drizzle with lemon juice, if using, and serve warm. Store in the fridge for up to 4 days.

Substitutions: Swap radishes for turnips; thyme for rosemary.

Why it Works: Radishes contain glucosinolates for immunity and DNA protection, while garlic boosts immune function. Olive oil supports microbiome health.

Citrus Sorbet (Dessert, no sugar)

Prep Time: 10 minutes
Cooking Time: 0 minutes (plus 4 hours freezing)
Total Time: 10 minutes active, 4 hours total
Servings: 4 (½ cup per serving, about 2 cups total)

Nutritional Information (per serving, ½ cup):

- Calories: 70 kcal
- Protein: 1 g
- Fat: 0 g
- Carbohydrates: 18 g (2 g fiber, 14 g sugar)
- Sodium: 0 mg

- Key Nutrients: Vitamin C (40% DV), Antioxidants (flavonoids)

Ingredients:

- 2 cups frozen orange segments (from 2–3 oranges)
- ½ cup frozen lemon segments (from 1 lemon, peeled)
- 1 tablespoon lemon juice
- 1 teaspoon orange zest

Instructions:

- Blend frozen orange and lemon segments, lemon juice, and orange zest in a food processor for 1–2 minutes until smooth.
- Serve as soft-serve or freeze in an airtight container for 2–4 hours for firmer texture. Let soften 5 minutes before scooping. Store in the freezer for up to 1 month.

Substitutions: Swap orange for grapefruit; lime for lemon.

Why it Works: Citrus fruits are rich in vitamin C and flavonoids, protecting DNA and inhibiting angiogenesis. This sorbet is a clean, no-sugar dessert aligned with Dr. Li's principles.

Creamy Broccoli Soup (Lunch, heart-healthy)

Prep Time: 10 minutes
Cooking Time: 20 minutes
Total Time: 30 minutes
Servings: 4 (1 cup per serving, about 4 cups total)

Nutritional Information (per serving, 1 cup):

- Calories: 160 kcal
- Protein: 5 g
- Fat: 10 g (1.5 g saturated)
- Carbohydrates: 14 g (4 g fiber, 3 g sugar)
- Sodium: 300 mg
- Key Nutrients: Vitamin C (50% DV), Vitamin K (30% DV)

Ingredients:

- 4 cups broccoli florets
- ½ cup raw cashews, soaked 4 hours and drained
- 1 small onion, chopped
- 1 garlic clove, minced
- 3 cups low-sodium vegetable broth
- 1 tablespoon olive oil
- ½ teaspoon salt
- ¼ teaspoon black pepper

Instructions:

- Sauté onion and garlic in olive oil in a saucepan over medium heat for 5 minutes.
- Add broccoli, cashews, broth, salt, and pepper. Simmer for 15 minutes until broccoli is tender.
- Blend until smooth with an immersion blender or in batches. Serve hot. Store in the fridge for up to 4 days.

Substitutions: Swap broccoli for cauliflower; almonds for cashews.

Why it Works: Broccoli's sulforaphane inhibits angiogenesis, while cashews support microbiome health. This soup is a clean, heart-healthy lunch aligned with Dr. Li's principles.

Lentil-Walnut Salad (Lunch, protein-packed)

Prep Time: 10 minutes
Cooking Time: 10 minutes (if cooking lentils)
Total Time: 20 minutes
Servings: 4 (1 cup per serving, about 4 cups total)

Nutritional Information (per serving, 1 cup):

- Calories: 240 kcal
- Protein: 12 g
- Fat: 12 g (1 g saturated)
- Carbohydrates: 24 g (8 g fiber, 2 g sugar)
- Sodium: 200 mg
- Key Nutrients: Fiber (32% DV), Iron (15% DV)

Ingredients:

- 2 cups cooked green lentils
- ½ cup walnuts, chopped
- 1 cup chopped celery
- 2 tablespoons olive oil
- 1 tablespoon red wine vinegar
- ½ teaspoon Dijon mustard
- ¼ teaspoon salt
- 2 tablespoons fresh parsley, chopped

Instructions:

- In a large bowl, combine lentils, walnuts, celery, olive oil, vinegar, mustard, salt, and parsley. Toss well.
- Serve immediately or chill for up to 4 hours. Store in the fridge for up to 4 days.

Substitutions: Swap lentils for chickpeas; pecans for walnuts.

Why it Works: Lentils provide prebiotic fiber for microbiome health, while walnuts offer omega-3s for angiogenesis inhibition. This salad is a clean, nutrient-dense lunch aligned with Dr. Li's principles.

Baked Cod with Tomato-Olive Relish

(Dinner)

Prep Time: 10 minutes
Cooking Time: 15 minutes
Total Time: 25 minutes
Servings: 4 (1 fillet per serving)

Nutritional Information (per serving, 1 fillet):

- Calories: 200 kcal
- Protein: 22 g
- Fat: 10 g (1.5 g saturated)
- Carbohydrates: 6 g (2 g fiber, 2 g sugar)
- Sodium: 300 mg
- Key Nutrients: Omega-3s (10% DV), Vitamin C (15% DV)

Ingredients:

- 4 cod fillets (4–5 oz each)
- 1 cup cherry tomatoes, halved
- ¼ cup pitted Kalamata olives, chopped
- 1 tablespoon olive oil
- 1 tablespoon lemon juice
- ½ teaspoon dried oregano
- ¼ teaspoon salt
- ¼ teaspoon black pepper

Instructions:

- Preheat oven to 400°F (200°C). Place cod in a parchment-lined baking dish, brush with ½ tablespoon olive oil, and season with salt and pepper.
- Bake for 12–15 minutes until fish flakes easily (145°F internal temperature).
- Mix tomatoes, olives, remaining olive oil, lemon juice, and oregano. Spoon over cod. Serve warm. Store in the fridge for up to 2 days.

Substitutions: Swap cod for haddock; capers for olives.

Why it Works: Cod provides omega-3s for angiogenesis inhibition, while tomatoes and olives support DNA protection.

Chapter 7: Immunity Warriors (Fighting Infections)

Ginger-Turmeric Tea

Prep Time: 5 minutes
Cooking Time: 5 minutes
Total Time: 10 minutes
Servings: 2

Nutritional Information (per serving):

- **Calories:** 20 kcal
- **Protein:** 0 g
- **Fat:** 0 g
- **Carbohydrates:** 5 g
- **Sodium:** 5 mg
- **Key Nutrients:** Antioxidants, anti-inflammatory compounds (Curcumin from turmeric), Vitamin C (from ginger)

Ingredients:

- 2 inches fresh ginger root (peeled and sliced)
- 1 teaspoon turmeric powder (or 1-inch fresh turmeric root)
- 2 cups water
- 1 tablespoon honey (optional)
- 1 tablespoon fresh lemon juice

Instructions:

1. **Boil Water:** In a small saucepan, bring 2 cups of water to a boil.
2. **Add Ginger and Turmeric:** Once boiling, add the fresh ginger and turmeric (or powdered turmeric). Reduce heat and simmer for 5 minutes.
3. **Strain and Sweeten:** Strain the liquid into two cups, then stir in honey and lemon juice to taste.
4. **Serve:** Serve hot and enjoy the warming, anti-inflammatory effects.

Substitutions:

- **Honey:** You can use maple syrup or agave syrup as alternatives.
- **Lemon:** If you don't have fresh lemons, a splash of apple cider vinegar can be used.

Serving Suggestions:
Enjoy with a side of nuts or fruit for a refreshing, immunity-boosting snack.

Why it Works:
Both ginger and turmeric are known for their anti-inflammatory properties and support immune health. This tea can help fight infections, reduce inflammation, and provide antioxidant benefits.

Garlic & Lemon Chicken Soup

Prep Time: 10 minutes
Cooking Time: 20 minutes
Total Time: 30 minutes
Servings: 4

Nutritional Information (per serving):

- **Calories:** 250 kcal
- **Protein:** 25 g
- **Fat:** 7 g
- **Carbohydrates:** 18 g
- **Sodium:** 500 mg
- **Key Nutrients:** Vitamin C (lemon), antioxidants (garlic), lean protein (chicken)

Ingredients:

- 2 chicken breasts (boneless, skinless)
- 6 cloves garlic (minced)
- 1 large onion (chopped)
- 2 carrots (sliced)
- 2 celery stalks (chopped)
- 4 cups chicken broth (low-sodium)
- 1 lemon (juiced)
- 1 teaspoon dried thyme
- Salt and pepper to taste
- 1 tablespoon olive oil

Instructions:

1. **Cook Chicken:** Heat olive oil in a large pot over medium heat. Add the chicken breasts and cook for 6-8 minutes per side, until fully cooked. Remove and set aside.
2. **Sauté Vegetables:** In the same pot, add garlic, onion, carrots, and celery. Sauté for 5 minutes, until softened.
3. **Add Broth:** Pour in chicken broth, thyme, and bring to a boil. Once boiling, reduce heat to simmer.
4. **Shred Chicken:** While the soup is simmering, shred the cooked chicken. Add it to the pot.
5. **Add Lemon and Season:** Stir in lemon juice and season with salt and pepper to taste.
6. **Simmer:** Let the soup simmer for an additional 10 minutes to blend the flavors.
7. **Serve:** Ladle soup into bowls and serve hot.

Substitutions:

- **Chicken:** You can use turkey or a plant-based protein like tofu for a vegetarian option.
- **Broth:** Vegetable broth can be used instead of chicken broth for a vegetarian version.

Serving Suggestions:
Serve with a side of whole grain crackers or a simple salad for added fiber.

Why it Works:
Garlic is known for its immune-boosting properties, and lemon provides a dose of Vitamin C. This soup is soothing and supportive for fighting infections.

Spinach and Kale Power Salad

Prep Time: 10 minutes
Cooking Time: 0 minutes
Total Time: 10 minutes
Servings: 4

Nutritional Information (per serving):

- **Calories:** 120 kcal
- **Protein:** 4 g
- **Fat:** 9 g
- **Carbohydrates:** 10 g
- **Sodium:** 150 mg
- **Key Nutrients:** Iron (spinach and kale), Vitamin K, antioxidants

Ingredients:

- 2 cups fresh spinach (washed)
- 2 cups fresh kale (washed and chopped)
- 1 avocado (sliced)
- ½ cup walnuts (chopped)
- 2 tablespoons olive oil
- 1 tablespoon apple cider vinegar
- Salt and pepper to taste

Instructions:

1. **Prepare Salad Base:** In a large bowl, combine spinach and kale.
2. **Add Toppings:** Top with sliced avocado, walnuts, and season with salt and pepper.
3. **Dress Salad:** In a small bowl, whisk together olive oil and apple cider vinegar. Drizzle the dressing over the salad.
4. **Serve:** Toss and serve immediately.

Substitutions:

- **Walnuts:** Swap walnuts for almonds, pecans, or seeds like pumpkin or sunflower.
- **Apple Cider Vinegar:** Lemon juice can be used as an alternative to vinegar.

Serving Suggestions:
Serve with a lean protein like grilled chicken or roasted chickpeas for a balanced meal.

Why it Works:
This salad combines nutrient-dense greens like spinach and kale, providing essential vitamins and antioxidants that support immune health. Walnuts offer healthy fats, while avocado adds a creamy texture.

Elderberry Syrup Smoothie

Prep Time: 5 minutes
Cooking Time: 0 minutes
Total Time: 5 minutes
Servings: 2

Nutritional Information (per serving):

- **Calories:** 200 kcal
- **Protein:** 3 g
- **Fat:** 6 g
- **Carbohydrates:** 34 g
- **Sodium:** 10 mg
- **Key Nutrients:** Antioxidants (elderberries), Vitamin C, fiber (from banana)

Ingredients:

- 1 tablespoon elderberry syrup
- 1 frozen banana
- ½ cup frozen mixed berries
- 1 cup unsweetened almond milk
- 1 tablespoon chia seeds (optional)

Instructions:

1. **Blend Ingredients:** In a blender, combine elderberry syrup, frozen banana, mixed berries, and almond milk.
2. **Add Chia Seeds:** Add chia seeds if using.
3. **Blend:** Blend until smooth.
4. **Serve:** Pour into glasses and serve immediately.

Substitutions:

- **Elderberry Syrup:** If you don't have elderberry syrup, you can try a homemade version or substitute with other immune-boosting ingredients like raw honey or lemon.
- **Almond Milk:** Any plant-based milk or dairy milk works as a substitute.

Serving Suggestions:
Enjoy as a quick breakfast or snack. Pair with a handful of nuts for an added protein boost.

Why it Works:
Elderberries are packed with antioxidants and have been shown to help reduce the severity and duration of cold and flu symptoms. This smoothie provides an immunity boost in a delicious, easy-to-consume form.

Miso Soup with Seaweed and Tofu

Prep Time: 5 minutes
Cooking Time: 10 minutes
Total Time: 15 minutes
Servings: 4

Nutritional Information (per serving):

- **Calories:** 100 kcal
- **Protein:** 8 g
- **Fat:** 5 g
- **Carbohydrates:** 10 g
- **Sodium:** 600 mg
- **Key Nutrients:** Probiotics (miso), protein (tofu), iodine (seaweed)

Ingredients:

- 2 tablespoons miso paste (white or yellow)
- 3 cups water
- 1 block firm tofu (cubed)
- 1 cup dried seaweed (wakame)
- 2 green onions (chopped)
- 1 tablespoon soy sauce (optional)

Instructions:

1. **Heat Broth:** In a small pot, combine water and miso paste. Heat over medium heat, whisking until the miso dissolves.
2. **Add Tofu & Seaweed:** Add cubed tofu and dried seaweed. Let it simmer for 5-7 minutes.
3. **Season:** Stir in soy sauce and green onions.
4. **Serve:** Ladle soup into bowls and serve hot.

Substitutions:

- **Tofu:** Tempeh or a plant-based protein like edamame can be used in place of tofu.
- **Seaweed:** You can skip seaweed or use spinach or kale for a leafy green option.

Serving Suggestions:

Pair with brown rice or a small salad for a complete meal.

Why it Works:
Miso is a fermented food that promotes gut health and immune function. The seaweed provides iodine, while tofu adds plant-based protein, making this soup a nourishing option for fighting infections.

Citrus and Berry Smoothie

Prep Time: 5 minutes
Cooking Time: 0 minutes
Total Time: 5 minutes
Servings: 2

Nutritional Information (per serving):

- **Calories:** 180 kcal
- **Protein:** 2 g
- **Fat:** 4 g
- **Carbohydrates:** 35 g
- **Sodium:** 10 mg
- **Key Nutrients:** Vitamin C (citrus and berries), antioxidants

Ingredients:

- 1 orange (peeled)
- 1 cup frozen mixed berries
- ½ cup Greek yogurt (optional)
- 1 tablespoon chia seeds
- 1 cup water or almond milk

Instructions:

1. **Blend Ingredients:** In a blender, combine orange, mixed berries, Greek yogurt (optional), chia seeds, and water/almond milk.
2. **Blend:** Blend until smooth.
3. **Serve:** Pour into glasses and serve immediately.

Substitutions:

- **Greek Yogurt:** You can use plant-based yogurt or skip it entirely for a dairy-free version.
- **Chia Seeds:** Flaxseeds or hemp seeds work as good alternatives.

Serving Suggestions:
Serve as a refreshing breakfast or snack with a handful of

nuts or a small granola bar for extra energy.

Why it Works:
Citrus fruits and berries are both packed with Vitamin C, which is essential for a healthy immune system. This smoothie is a delicious and refreshing way to get your daily dose of antioxidants.

Fermented Kimchi with Brown Rice

Prep Time: 10 minutes
Cooking Time: 0 minutes (fermentation time required)
Total Time: 1-2 weeks (fermentation)
Servings: 4

Nutritional Information (per serving):

- **Calories:** 150 kcal
- **Protein:** 4 g
- **Fat:** 5 g
- **Carbohydrates:** 24 g
- **Sodium:** 500 mg
- **Key Nutrients:** Probiotics (kimchi), fiber (brown rice), Vitamin A and C (kimchi)

Ingredients:

- 1 cup kimchi (fermented)
- 2 cups cooked brown rice
- 1 tablespoon sesame oil
- 1 tablespoon sesame seeds
- 2 green onions (chopped)

Instructions:

1. **Prepare Brown Rice:** Cook 2 cups of brown rice as per package instructions.
2. **Combine Kimchi and Rice:** Once the rice is cooked and cooled, mix in the fermented kimchi.
3. **Add Flavor:** Drizzle sesame oil over the mixture and toss in sesame seeds and chopped green onions.
4. **Serve:** Serve immediately or store in the fridge to allow the flavors to meld further.

Substitutions:

- **Sesame Oil:** Can be substituted with olive oil or avocado oil for a lighter option.
- **Kimchi:** Use sauerkraut or another fermented vegetable if kimchi isn't available.

Serving Suggestions:
Pair this dish with a side of steamed vegetables or grilled chicken for added protein.

Why it Works:
Kimchi is a probiotic powerhouse that supports gut health and the immune system, while brown rice provides fiber and steady energy, making this dish perfect for overall health and immunity.

Roasted Garlic and Broccoli

Prep Time: 10 minutes
Cooking Time: 20 minutes
Total Time: 30 minutes
Servings: 4

Nutritional Information (per serving):

- **Calories:** 100 kcal
- **Protein:** 4 g
- **Fat:** 7 g
- **Carbohydrates:** 12 g
- **Sodium:** 25 mg
- **Key Nutrients:** Antioxidants (garlic), Vitamin C (broccoli), healthy fats (olive oil)

Ingredients:

- 2 cups broccoli florets
- 6 garlic cloves (minced)
- 2 tablespoons olive oil
- Salt and pepper to taste
- 1 tablespoon lemon juice (optional)

Instructions:

1. **Preheat Oven:** Preheat your oven to 400°F (200°C).
2. **Toss Broccoli and Garlic:** In a large mixing bowl, toss broccoli florets and minced garlic with olive oil, salt, and pepper.
3. **Roast:** Spread the mixture onto a baking sheet in a single layer. Roast for 20 minutes, tossing halfway through.
4. **Serve:** Once golden and tender, drizzle with lemon juice (optional) and serve.

Substitutions:

- **Olive Oil:** Can be replaced with avocado oil or melted coconut oil.
- **Lemon Juice:** A splash of apple cider vinegar can also work for an extra zing.

Serving Suggestions:
Serve as a side dish with grilled meats or roasted tofu for a nutrient-dense meal.

Why it Works:
Garlic is a powerful immune booster, while broccoli provides Vitamin C and antioxidants to support overall health and fight infections.

Chia Seed Pudding with Turmeric and Honey

Prep Time: 5 minutes
Cooking Time: 0 minutes
Total Time: 4 hours (overnight for best results)
Servings: 2

Nutritional Information (per serving):

- **Calories:** 220 kcal
- **Protein:** 5 g
- **Fat:** 12 g
- **Carbohydrates:** 20 g
- **Sodium:** 10 mg
- **Key Nutrients:** Omega-3 (chia seeds), anti-inflammatory (turmeric), antioxidants (honey)

Ingredients:

- 3 tablespoons chia seeds
- 1 cup almond milk (or any milk of choice)
- 1 teaspoon turmeric powder
- 1 tablespoon honey
- 1 teaspoon vanilla extract (optional)

Instructions:

1. **Mix Ingredients:** In a bowl, combine chia seeds, almond milk, turmeric powder, honey, and vanilla extract (if using).
2. **Refrigerate:** Stir well and refrigerate for at least 4 hours or overnight to allow the chia seeds to absorb the liquid and thicken.
3. **Serve:** Serve chilled, garnished with extra honey or fruit if desired.

Substitutions:

- **Honey:** Maple syrup or agave can be used for a vegan option.
- **Almond Milk:** Any milk (dairy or plant-based) works fine.

Serving Suggestions:
Top with fresh fruit like berries, mango, or a sprinkle of cinnamon for extra flavor and nutrition.

Why it Works:
Chia seeds are rich in omega-3 fatty acids, which reduce inflammation, while turmeric has powerful anti-inflammatory properties. This pudding is a great snack or breakfast option to support immune health.

Carrot & Ginger Immunity Juice

Prep Time: 5 minutes
Cooking Time: 0 minutes
Total Time: 5 minutes
Servings: 2

Nutritional Information (per serving):

- **Calories:** 150 kcal
- **Protein:** 1 g
- **Fat:** 0 g
- **Carbohydrates:** 36 g
- **Sodium:** 60 mg
- **Key Nutrients:** Vitamin A (carrots), antioxidants (ginger), Vitamin C

Ingredients:

- 4 large carrots (peeled)
- 1-inch piece fresh ginger (peeled)
- 1 lemon (peeled)
- 1 tablespoon honey (optional)
- 1 cup water or coconut water

Instructions:

1. **Juice Ingredients:** In a juicer, combine carrots, ginger, and lemon.
2. **Add Liquid:** Add the water or coconut water to dilute to desired consistency.
3. **Serve:** Pour into glasses and add honey if you prefer a sweeter taste.

Substitutions:

- **Honey:** Maple syrup or agave syrup works well as a substitute.
- **Coconut Water:** Plain water or almond water can be used.

Serving Suggestions:
Pair this juice with a light breakfast like oatmeal or a piece of whole-grain toast for a balanced morning meal.

Why it Works:
Carrots are packed with beta-carotene (Vitamin A) for immune support, while ginger provides anti-inflammatory properties that help fight infections. This juice is refreshing and nourishing for your immune system.

Chicken and Mushroom Stir Fry

Prep Time: 10 minutes
Cooking Time: 15 minutes
Total Time: 25 minutes
Servings: 4

Nutritional Information (per serving):

- **Calories:** 300 kcal
- **Protein:** 30 g
- **Fat:** 12 g
- **Carbohydrates:** 15 g
- **Sodium:** 500 mg

- **Key Nutrients:** Lean protein (chicken), antioxidants (mushrooms), Vitamin B (mushrooms)

Ingredients:

- 2 chicken breasts (sliced thinly)
- 2 cups mushrooms (sliced)
- 1 onion (sliced)
- 2 tablespoons olive oil
- 2 tablespoons soy sauce (low-sodium)
- 1 teaspoon sesame oil
- 2 cloves garlic (minced)
- 1 tablespoon fresh ginger (grated)
- Salt and pepper to taste

Instructions:

1. **Cook Chicken:** Heat olive oil in a large pan over medium heat. Add chicken and cook until browned, about 6-8 minutes. Remove and set aside.
2. **Sauté Veggies:** In the same pan, add mushrooms, onion, garlic, and ginger. Cook for 5 minutes, until mushrooms are soft.
3. **Combine:** Add chicken back to the pan and pour in soy sauce and sesame oil. Stir well to coat.
4. **Serve:** Season with salt and pepper to taste, then serve immediately.

Substitutions:

- **Chicken:** You can use turkey, tofu, or tempeh for a vegetarian version.
- **Soy Sauce:** Coconut aminos or tamari can be used as soy sauce alternatives.

Serving Suggestions:
Serve this stir-fry with a side of quinoa or brown rice for a well-rounded meal.

Why it Works:
Chicken provides lean protein for tissue repair and immune function, while mushrooms contain beta-glucans, which help activate immune cells. This stir-fry is packed with flavor and supports immune health.

Apple Cider Vinegar Detox Drink

Prep Time: 2 minutes
Cooking Time: 0 minutes
Total Time: 2 minutes
Servings: 1

Nutritional Information (per serving):

- **Calories:** 10 kcal
- **Protein:** 0 g
- **Fat:** 0 g
- **Carbohydrates:** 2 g
- **Sodium:** 5 mg
- **Key Nutrients:** Detoxifying properties (apple cider vinegar), probiotics

Ingredients:

- 1 tablespoon apple cider vinegar
- 1 cup warm water
- 1 teaspoon honey (optional)
- 1 teaspoon lemon juice (optional)

Instructions:

1. **Mix:** Combine the apple cider vinegar, warm water, and optional honey and lemon juice in a glass. Stir well.
2. **Serve:** Drink immediately, preferably before meals.

Substitutions:

- **Honey:** Maple syrup or stevia can be used as a substitute.
- **Lemon Juice:** Lime juice can be used as an alternative.

Serving Suggestions:
This detox drink can be consumed daily before meals or as a refreshing morning routine.

Why it Works:
Apple cider vinegar helps balance the body's pH and supports digestion, while lemon juice provides a boost of Vitamin C to enhance immunity.

Roasted Butternut Squash Soup

Prep Time: 15 minutes
Cooking Time: 40 minutes
Total Time: 55 minutes
Servings: 4

Nutritional Information (per serving):

- **Calories:** 200 kcal
- **Protein:** 3 g
- **Fat:** 8 g
- **Carbohydrates:** 32 g
- **Sodium:** 300 mg
- **Key Nutrients:** Vitamin A (butternut squash), fiber, antioxidants

Ingredients:

- 1 medium butternut squash (peeled, seeded, cubed)
- 1 small onion (chopped)
- 2 cloves garlic (minced)
- 1 tablespoon olive oil
- 4 cups vegetable broth
- 1 teaspoon ground cinnamon
- 1/2 teaspoon ground nutmeg
- Salt and pepper to taste
- 1/2 cup coconut milk (optional for creaminess)

Instructions:

1. **Roast Squash:** Preheat oven to 400°F (200°C). Toss squash cubes with olive oil, salt, and pepper. Spread on a baking sheet and roast for 25–30 minutes until tender.

2. **Sauté Aromatics:** In a large pot, sauté onion and garlic until translucent.

3. **Simmer:** Add roasted squash, broth, cinnamon, and nutmeg. Bring to a simmer for 10 minutes.

4. **Blend:** Use an immersion blender (or carefully transfer to a regular blender) to purée until smooth.

5. **Finish:** Stir in coconut milk (if using) for extra creaminess. Adjust seasoning as needed.

6. **Serve:** Garnish with a swirl of coconut milk or a sprinkle of pumpkin seeds.

Substitutions:

- **Coconut Milk:** Can be replaced with regular cream, almond milk, or omitted entirely.
- **Butternut Squash:** Substitute with sweet potatoes or pumpkin.

Serving Suggestions:
Pair with a slice of crusty whole-grain bread or a light salad for a complete meal.

Why it Works:
Butternut squash is loaded with immune-supporting Vitamin A and antioxidants, while the warming spices boost circulation and digestion—perfect for cold season protection!

Zinc-Rich Pumpkin Seed Pesto

Prep Time: 10 minutes
Cooking Time: 0 minutes
Total Time: 10 minutes
Servings: 6 (about 2 tablespoons per serving)

Nutritional Information (per serving):

- **Calories:** 110 kcal
- **Protein:** 4 g
- **Fat:** 10 g
- **Carbohydrates:** 2 g
- **Sodium:** 100 mg
- **Key Nutrients:** Zinc (pumpkin seeds), healthy fats, antioxidants

Ingredients:

- 1/2 cup pumpkin seeds (pepitas)
- 1 cup fresh basil leaves
- 1/4 cup olive oil
- 2 tablespoons nutritional yeast (or Parmesan cheese)
- 2 cloves garlic
- Juice of 1/2 lemon
- Salt and pepper to taste

Instructions:

1. **Toast Seeds:** Lightly toast pumpkin seeds in a dry skillet over medium heat until fragrant (about 3 minutes), stirring often.

2. **Blend:** In a food processor, combine pumpkin seeds, basil, olive oil, nutritional yeast, garlic, and lemon juice. Blend until smooth.

3. **Season:** Add salt and pepper to taste. Blend again briefly to mix.

4. **Store:** Keep in an airtight container in the fridge for up to a week.

Substitutions:

- **Pumpkin Seeds:** Sunflower seeds or walnuts can be used.
- **Nutritional Yeast:** Parmesan cheese if dairy is fine for you.

Serving Suggestions:
Use as a spread on sandwiches, a sauce for pasta or roasted veggies, or as a dip for crackers.

Why it Works:
Pumpkin seeds are one of the best natural sources of zinc, a crucial mineral for immune function. Combined with antioxidant-rich basil, this pesto is as powerful as it is delicious!

Lentil & Tomato Soup with Spinach

Prep Time: 10 minutes
Cooking Time: 35 minutes
Total Time: 45 minutes
Servings: 4

Nutritional Information (per serving):

- **Calories:** 250 kcal
- **Protein:** 15 g
- **Fat:** 4 g
- **Carbohydrates:** 38 g
- **Sodium:** 400 mg
- **Key Nutrients:** Plant protein (lentils), Vitamin C (tomatoes), iron (spinach)

Ingredients:

- 1 cup dried brown or green lentils (rinsed)
- 1 can (15 oz) diced tomatoes
- 4 cups vegetable broth
- 1 small onion (chopped)
- 2 cloves garlic (minced)
- 1 teaspoon cumin
- 1 teaspoon smoked paprika
- 2 cups fresh spinach leaves
- 1 tablespoon olive oil

- Salt and pepper to taste

Instructions:

1. **Sauté Aromatics:** Heat olive oil in a large pot. Sauté onion and garlic until translucent.
2. **Add Lentils and Tomatoes:** Stir in lentils, canned tomatoes (with juice), cumin, and paprika.
3. **Simmer:** Pour in broth and bring to a boil. Reduce heat and simmer for 30–35 minutes until lentils are tender.
4. **Finish with Spinach:** Stir in spinach and cook just until wilted (about 2–3 minutes).
5. **Season:** Adjust salt and pepper to taste before serving.

Substitutions:

- **Spinach:** Swap with kale or Swiss chard if preferred.
- **Canned Tomatoes:** Use fresh chopped tomatoes when in season.

Serving Suggestions:
Enjoy with a drizzle of olive oil or a sprinkle of chili flakes for extra warmth. Add a side of whole-grain bread for a hearty meal.

Why it Works:
Lentils deliver protein and iron, critical for strong immunity, while tomatoes and spinach provide antioxidants and Vitamin C to boost defense mechanisms naturally.

Tips for Success

Bringing Your Recipes to Life

Cooking isn't just about following a recipe word for word — it's about *bringing food to life* with attention, intuition, and a little creativity.

When you understand *how* to approach a recipe — not just *what* to do — you unlock a whole new level of ease and confidence in the kitchen.

Whether you're making a vibrant immunity-boosting soup, a DNA-defense smoothie, or a cozy batch-cooked stew, **these key tips will ensure your recipes shine** — and your cooking experience feels joyful, not stressful.

1. Read the Entire Recipe Before You Start

This may seem obvious, but it's one of the most powerful secrets of successful cooking. Reading through the full recipe — ingredients, instructions, notes, and suggestions — gives you:

- A clear roadmap of what's coming
- A sense of timing for different steps
- Insight into any special techniques (like "simmer gently" or "fold carefully")

You'll avoid surprises, and your flow in the kitchen will be smoother and more confident.

Pro Tip: Mentally picture the steps as you read. This tiny habit boosts memory and minimizes mistakes.

2. Prep Your Ingredients First (a.k.a. Mise en Place)

Mise en place is a French culinary phrase that means "everything in its place." Before you turn on the stove, **wash, chop, measure, and organize all your ingredients**.

Why it matters:

- Prevents frantic last-minute measuring while something is burning
- Helps you spot if you're missing anything *before* you start
- Makes cooking feel calm, focused, and even meditative

Think of it as setting the stage for a beautiful performance — you're the star chef!

3. Use Fresh, High-Quality Ingredients

Especially when you're cooking for health — boosting immunity, fighting inflammation, or supporting DNA repair — the quality of your ingredients matters. Fresh produce, high-quality oils, vibrant herbs, and good proteins *taste better* and *nourish deeper*.

If you can:

- Choose seasonal and organic when possible.
- Visit farmers' markets for ultra-fresh finds.
- Look for "alive" foods: bright greens, fragrant herbs, rich-colored berries.

Remember: The more alive your food is, the more it gives life back to you.

4. Taste As You Go

The best chefs taste constantly during cooking — and you should too! Adjust seasoning little by little (salt, acid, herbs, spices) to balance the flavors.

Tasting transforms a good meal into a great one because:

- Different vegetables vary in sweetness and bitterness
- Spices and herbs lose potency over time
- Cooking methods (like roasting) can concentrate or mellow flavors

Trust your palate. Recipes are a starting point; your tastebuds guide the final masterpiece.

5. Respect Heat and Timing

Every recipe includes heat and time not as random suggestions but as a science of flavor and texture.

- **Too high heat?** You risk burning delicate ingredients or drying out meat.
- **Too low heat?** You might end up with mushy vegetables or bland, watery dishes.

Learn to recognize *visual* and *sensory* cues:

- Simmering means gentle bubbling (not vigorous boiling).
- Golden-brown roasting often smells nutty and sweet.
- Stir-fries should sizzle with life but not smoke excessively.

Tip: Use a kitchen timer when needed, but also trust your eyes, nose, and intuition.

6. Stay Flexible and Adapt

Ingredients, kitchen tools, and even your daily mood can vary.
A recipe is a map — not a cage.

Feel free to adjust based on:

- What you have on hand (sub spinach for kale, or brown rice for quinoa)
- Your taste preferences (more spice? extra lemon?)
- Dietary needs (gluten-free swaps, dairy alternatives)

Some of the most delicious dishes are born from happy improvisation!

7. Presentation Matters (Because You Eat With Your Eyes First!)

How you plate your food influences how much you enjoy it.
Simple, colorful garnishes — a sprinkle of chopped herbs, a drizzle of sauce, a twist of lemon — elevate even the simplest dishes into a feast.

Easy tricks:

- Use white or neutral plates to let colors pop.
- Add a sprinkle of seeds, nuts, or microgreens for texture.
- Wipe plate edges clean for a polished finish.

Cooking is an act of love — and beautiful presentation makes it even more special.

8. Celebrate Small Wins

Each time you try a new recipe, master a new technique, or discover a flavor you love — *celebrate it*!
Cooking is a skill built with time, patience, and joy.

Every meal is a chance to nurture yourself and your loved ones.

Even if a dish isn't "perfect," you learned something valuable — and that's success worth savoring.

Recipes are not rules; they are invitations — invitations to nourish yourself, to connect with your senses, to create something beautiful with your own hands. When you approach cooking with curiosity, care, and a little courage, every meal becomes an act of wellness and creativity.

The real tip for success? Bring your heart to the table.
The rest will follow.

Chapter 8: 30 Day Meal Plan

Week 1

Day 1:

- Breakfast: Blueberry-Spinach Smoothie
- Lunch: Roasted Tomato Soup + Pumpkin Seed Crackers
- Dinner: Grilled Salmon with Raspberry Salsa
- Snack: Maple-Walnut Granola

Day 2:

- Breakfast: Banana-Oat Muffins
- Lunch: Tuna Quinoa Bowl
- Dinner: Sweet Potato and Black Bean Tacos
- Dessert: Berry-Coconut Popsicles

Day 3:

- Breakfast: Cocoa-Banana Smoothie
- Lunch: Apple-Walnut Salad
- Dinner: Olive Oil Poached Cod
- Snack: Garlic-Herb Roasted Chickpeas

Day 4:

- Breakfast: Kale-Avocado Breakfast Bowl (With Poached Egg)
- Lunch: Pomegranate-Glazed Carrots + Roasted Parsnips with Thyme
- Dinner: Lentil-Pumpkin Stew
- Dessert: Dark Chocolate-Oat Bites

Day 5:

- Breakfast: Spinach and Mushroom Frittata
- Lunch: Strawberry-Arugula Salad
- Dinner: Turmeric-Ginger Roasted Cauliflower Steaks
- Snack: Berry-Chia Jam on Almond-Oat Flatbread

Day 6:

- Breakfast: Golden Turmeric Quinoa
- Lunch: Beet Hummus with Pumpkin Seed Crackers
- Dinner: Tuna-Stuffed Bell Peppers
- Dessert: Red Grape Sorbet

Day 7:

- Breakfast: Coconut-Cashew Yogurt with Maple-Walnut Granola
- Lunch: Roasted Tomato Soup + Shiitake and Spinach Soup
- Dinner: Bok Choy & Tofu Stir Fry
- Snack: Almond Butter Cups

Week 2

Day 8:

- Breakfast: Cocoa-Banana Smoothie
- Lunch: Sweet Potato and Kale Hash
- Dinner: Black Garlic Roasted Chicken
- Dessert: Fig and Almond Tart

Day 9:
- Breakfast: Kale-Avocado Breakfast Bowl
- Lunch: Broccoli-Avocado Salad
- Dinner: Wild Mushroom Stir Fry
- Snack: Kale Chips

Day 10:
- Breakfast: Avocado-Chickpea Pita
- Lunch: Lentil-Walnut Salad
- Dinner: Grilled Salmon with Broccoli Salsa
- Dessert: Citrus Sorbet

Day 11:
- Breakfast: Maple-Walnut Granola with Coconut-Cashew Yogurt
- Lunch: Tomato-Walnut Bruschetta
- Dinner: Oyster Mushroom Tacos
- Snack: Carrot & Ginger Immunity Juice

Day 12:
- Breakfast: Turmeric Tea Latte + Banana-Oat Muffin
- Lunch: Cabbage and Apple Stir-Fry
- Dinner: Baked Cod with Tomato-Olive Relish
- Dessert: Cinnamon-Roasted Pears

Day 13:
- Breakfast: Spinach and Kale Power Salad (hearty breakfast salad!)
- Lunch: Garlic & Lemon Chicken Soup
- Dinner: Cauliflower Steaks with Tahini
- Snack: Chia Seed Pudding with Turmeric and Honey

Day 14:
- Breakfast: Coconut-Cashew Yogurt with Berry-Chia Jam
- Lunch: Zucchini Ribbon Salad with Lemon-Pepper Dressing
- Dinner: Chicken and Mushroom Stir Fry
- Snack: Cocoa-Hazelnut Spread on Chickpea Flour Tortillas

Week 3

Day 15:
- Breakfast: Citrus and Berry Smoothie
- Lunch: Miso Soup with Seaweed and Tofu
- Dinner: Sweet Potato and Black Bean Tacos
- Dessert: Orange-Zest Chia Pudding

Day 16:
- Breakfast: Golden Turmeric Quinoa
- Lunch: Roasted Radishes with Garlic + Roasted Garlic and Broccoli
- Dinner: Lentil & Tomato Soup with Spinach
- Snack: Zinc-Rich Pumpkin Seed Pesto with Crackers

Day 17:
- Breakfast: Cocoa-Banana Smoothie
- Lunch: Pomegranate-Glazed Carrots
- Dinner: Baked Sweet Potato with Tahini Drizzle
- Dessert: Red Grape Sorbet

Day 18:
- Breakfast: Berry-Coconut Popsicles (light morning)
- Lunch: Apple-Walnut Salad
- Dinner: Turmeric Chicken Skillet
- Snack: Carrot & Ginger Immunity Juice

Day 19:
- Breakfast: Elderberry Syrup Smoothie
- Lunch: Cabbage and Apple Stir-Fry
- Dinner: Lentil & Eggplant Shepherd's Pie
- Snack: Almond Butter Cups

Day 20:
- Breakfast: Chia Seed Pudding with Turmeric and Honey
- Lunch: Creamy Broccoli Soup
- Dinner: Bok Choy & Tofu Stir Fry
- Dessert: Dark Chocolate-Oat Bites

Day 21:
- Breakfast: Coconut-Cashew Yogurt with Maple-Walnut Granola
- Lunch: Tomato-Walnut Bruschetta
- Dinner: Olive Oil Poached Cod
- Snack: Fermented Kimchi with Brown Rice

Week 4

Day 22:
- Breakfast: Turmeric Tea Latte + Banana-Oat Muffins
- Lunch: Spinach and Kale Power Salad
- Dinner: Oyster Mushroom Tacos
- Dessert: Orange-Zest Chia Pudding

Day 23:
- Breakfast: Golden Turmeric Quinoa
- Lunch: Roasted Tomato Soup
- Dinner: Cauliflower Steaks with Pesto
- Snack: Garlic-Herb Roasted Chickpeas

Day 24:
- Breakfast: Berry-Coconut Popsicles
- Lunch: Broccoli-Avocado Salad
- Dinner: Black Garlic Roasted Chicken
- Dessert: Cinnamon-Roasted Pears

Day 25:
- Breakfast: Cocoa-Banana Smoothie
- Lunch: Brussels Sprouts with Pomegranate
- Dinner: Grilled Mackerel with Citrus
- Snack: Roasted Garlic and Broccoli

Day 26:

- Breakfast: Coconut-Cashew Yogurt with Maple-Walnut Granola
- Lunch: Tomato-Walnut Bruschetta
- Dinner: Garlic & Lemon Chicken Soup
- Dessert: Fig and Almond Tart

Day 27:

- Breakfast: Spinach and Mushroom Frittata
- Lunch: Apple-Walnut Salad
- Dinner: Shiitake and Spinach Soup
- Snack: Carrot & Ginger Immunity Juice

Day 28:

- Breakfast: Avocado-Chickpea Pita
- Lunch: Lentil-Walnut Salad
- Dinner: Baked Cod with Tomato-Olive Relish
- Dessert: Citrus Sorbet

Day 29:

- Breakfast: Cocoa-Hazelnut Spread on Almond-Oat Flatbread
- Lunch: Zucchini Ribbon Salad with Lemon-Pepper Dressing
- Dinner: Chicken and Mushroom Stir Fry
- Snack: Kale Chips

Day 30:

- Breakfast: Blueberry-Spinach Smoothie
- Lunch: Cabbage and Apple Stir-Fry
- Dinner: Grilled Salmon with Raspberry Salsa
- Dessert: Berry-Coconut Popsicles

shopping list

Vegetables

- Spinach (fresh & frozen if needed)
- Kale
- Arugula
- Broccoli (florets + stems)
- Cauliflower
- Brussels sprouts
- Zucchini
- Sweet potatoes
- Carrots
- Beets
- Radishes
- Bell peppers (green, red, yellow)
- Bok choy
- Shiitake mushrooms
- Oyster mushrooms
- Cremini or button mushrooms
- Garlic
- Onions (red + yellow)
- Scallions (green onions)
- Parsnips
- Cabbage (red + green)
- Avocados
- Tomatoes (cherry + large)
- Grape tomatoes
- Lemons
- Limes
- Ginger
- Fresh turmeric root
- Cilantro
- Fresh parsley
- Thyme
- Basil
- Pomegranate (or seeds)
- Olives (Kalamata or black)

Fruits

- Bananas
- Apples (green + red)
- Blueberries (fresh/frozen)
- Strawberries
- Raspberries
- Blackberries
- Red grapes
- Oranges
- Pears
- Citrus mix (orange, lemon, lime, grapefruit)
- Figs (fresh or dried)
- Elderberries (fresh/frozen or dried for syrup)

Nuts & Seeds

- Walnuts
- Almonds
- Cashews (raw)
- Pumpkin seeds (pepitas)
- Chia seeds
- Flaxseeds
- Sunflower seeds
- Hazelnuts

Legumes & Grains

- Chickpeas (canned or dried)
- Lentils (brown + red)
- Quinoa
- Brown rice
- Rolled oats
- Whole grain flatbread or tortillas (chickpea flour optional)
- Almond flour or oat flour (for flatbreads/muffins)
- Coconut flour (optional)

Pantry Essentials

- Extra virgin olive oil
- Coconut oil
- Avocado oil
- Apple cider vinegar
- Balsamic vinegar
- Tamari or low-sodium soy sauce
- Miso paste
- Dijon mustard
- Maple syrup
- Honey (local/raw if possible)
- Sea salt / Himalayan pink salt
- Black pepper
- Cumin
- Smoked paprika
- Ground cinnamon
- Turmeric (dried)
- Curry powder
- Chili flakes
- Garlic powder
- Onion powder
- Nutritional yeast
- Vegetable broth (low-sodium)
- Tomato paste
- Canned tomatoes
- Seaweed (nori or wakame)
- Baking soda/powder (for muffins)

Frozen Foods

- Frozen blueberries
- Frozen mixed berries

- Frozen spinach or kale (optional for smoothies)
- Frozen elderberries (or dried)

Proteins (Plant-Based + Optional Animal-Based)

- Tofu (firm or extra firm)
- Tempeh (optional)
- Canned tuna or salmon (wild-caught)
- Cod (fresh or frozen, or substitute with a white fish)
- Salmon fillets
- Chicken breast or thighs (pasture-raised if possible)
- Eggs (pastured, organic if possible)

Dairy Alternatives & Extras

- Unsweetened coconut yogurt or cashew yogurt
- Nut milk (almond, oat, cashew)
- Dark chocolate (70%+ cacao, optional for bites)
- Coconut cream or full-fat coconut milk
- Cocoa powder (unsweetened)

Fermented/Probiotic-Rich

- Kimchi
- Sauerkraut
- Coconut kefir or vegan yogurt with live cultures

How to Stick to Dr. Li's Diet Without Feeling Overwhelmed

Changing how you eat — even when it's for exciting reasons like boosting your immunity, protecting your DNA, or feeling more energized — can feel a little *overwhelming* at first.
That's completely normal. **Big changes are built from small, manageable steps.**

Here's how to make Dr. Li's diet second nature without stressing yourself out:

1. Start Simple. Focus on Adding, Not Restricting.

Instead of focusing on everything you *shouldn't* eat, **focus on adding more foods that support your body's defense systems** — berries, greens, nuts, seafood, colorful vegetables, fermented foods, etc.
Ask yourself: *What can I ADD to this meal that will help my body thrive?*

Even just tossing spinach into a sandwich or adding walnuts to your oatmeal counts as progress.

2. Master a Few Core Recipes First

You don't need to cook fancy meals every night.
Pick 3–5 recipes from this book that sound easy and delicious.
Make them a few times until they feel second nature.

Example: A simple Berry-Spinach Smoothie, Garlic-Herb Roasted Chickpeas, and Roasted Tomato Soup could become your go-to staples.

Once those feel easy, you can explore more recipes.

3. Prep Once, Eat Well All Week

Meal prepping even **one or two components** can change everything.

- Make a **batch of quinoa** or **Golden Turmeric Quinoa** for easy bowls.
- Roast a **sheet pan of veggies** (like cauliflower, carrots, mushrooms).
- Blend a jar of **Berry-Chia Jam** for quick breakfasts and snacks.
- Make a **big pot of soup** (like Shiitake and Spinach Soup) to reheat.

Having building blocks ready makes sticking to the diet effortless.

4. Plan Your Meals — Lightly

You don't have to micromanage every bite, but knowing a few meals in advance removes so much stress.
Try setting a simple **weekly plan** like:

- 2 quick breakfasts
- 2 lunches you can pack or reheat
- 2 dinners you're excited about
- 1 or 2 "flexible" snacks (like hummus + veggies)

A light plan means fewer last-minute decisions = less overwhelm.

5. Allow for Flexibility and Imperfection

You don't need to be perfect to see benefits.
If you eat a pizza on a busy Friday night, you didn't "fail" — you're living.
Just come back to nourishing foods at your next meal.
Consistency matters more than perfection.

6. Use Shortcuts When You Need Them

No time to cook lentils? Buy pre-cooked ones.
Don't want to roast beets? Get them ready-to-eat from the produce section.
Frozen berries, canned beans, and pre-washed greens are absolutely allowed.

Your health journey should *support* your life, not complicate it.

7. Celebrate Every Win

Every smoothie you blend, every vegetable you roast, every mindful meal you eat — it matters.
Celebrate small successes.
Success is built through hundreds of small, loving choices stacked over time.

Favorite Meal Prep Hacks for Dr. Li's Diet

Prepping smart saves you time, energy, and helps you eat defense-system-boosting foods all week without thinking about it.

Here are some tried hacks:

1. Batch Cook Breakfasts

- **Berry-Chia Jam:** Prep a jar and use it all week.
- **Banana-Oat Muffins:** Bake a dozen and freeze for grab-and-go mornings.
- **Coconut-Cashew Yogurt:** Make a batch for parfaits or snacks.

2. Double Up Dinners

Cook extra portions of:

- Roasted Cauliflower Steaks
- Lentil-Pumpkin Stew
- Grilled Salmon with Broccoli Salsa
  Eat one serving fresh, and pack the rest for easy lunches.

3. Use a "Magic Bowl" Formula

Keep cooked quinoa, roasted veggies, and greens on hand.
Throw in whatever is handy + a drizzle of dressing = Instant meal!
Example: Quinoa + kale + roasted mushrooms + olive oil + lemon.

4. Soup Is Your Best Friend

Soups like Miso Soup with Seaweed and Tofu or Roasted Tomato Soup reheat beautifully and are packed with defense-boosting ingredients.
Make a big pot once a week.

5. Smart Shopping = Easy Week

When you shop, think:

- 2 fruits (e.g., berries, apples)
- 2 greens (e.g., spinach, kale)
- 2 proteins (e.g., salmon, chickpeas)
- 2 grains (e.g., quinoa, oats)
- 2 extras (e.g., walnuts, dark chocolate)

You'll always have basics to throw together meals without a full recipe.

6. Pre-Wash and Prep Produce Right Away

As soon as you get home from the store:

- Wash berries and greens
- Chop carrots and celery
- Portion nuts and seeds into small bags

Future-you will be so thankful.

7. Theme Nights Make It Easy

- Monday = Salad night (Spinach and Kale Power Salad)

- Tuesday = Tacos (Oyster Mushroom Tacos)
- Wednesday = Soup night
- Thursday = Stir fry (Bok Choy and Tofu)
- Friday = Grilled fish night (Salmon, Mackerel)

Themes reduce decision fatigue and keep things fun.

Eating for health should make your life *easier and more joyful,* not harder. These small systems will help you stay consistent, stay energized, and feel amazing — one delicious bite at a time.

20 burning questions and answers for beginners

1. What exactly is Dr. Li's diet, and how does it work?

Answer: Dr. Li's diet is based on the concept of using food as medicine to promote long-term health and prevent disease. It focuses on eating foods that support angiogenesis (the growth of healthy blood vessels) and the microbiome, emphasizing whole, plant-based foods rich in antioxidants, healthy fats, and fiber.

2. Can I still eat meat on Dr. Li's diet?

Answer: Dr. Li's diet primarily promotes plant-based foods. While small amounts of animal protein are not entirely excluded, it encourages minimizing animal products to optimize health benefits and support angiogenesis and gut health.

3. Is this diet suitable for someone who has never been plant-based?

Answer: Yes, absolutely! Dr. Li's diet is adaptable for beginners and does not require an immediate switch to full plant-based eating. Start gradually by incorporating more plant-based meals and reducing processed foods and animal products over time.

4. How do I get enough protein on Dr. Li's diet?

Answer: Protein can be easily obtained from plant-based sources like legumes (lentils, chickpeas), beans, tofu, tempeh, nuts, seeds, and whole grains. Dr. Li's diet includes high-protein plant foods to ensure you meet your daily needs.

5. Can I drink coffee or alcohol on Dr. Li's diet?

Answer: Dr. Li suggests minimizing or avoiding alcohol and caffeine as much as possible, as they can disrupt the microbiome and affect your overall health. However, occasional consumption in moderation is fine.

6. Are there any foods I should completely avoid?

Answer: Yes, processed foods, refined sugars, artificial additives, and trans fats should be avoided. Dr. Li recommends minimizing highly processed items that can negatively impact your health and the growth of healthy blood vessels.

7. How do I start Dr. Li's diet if I'm a beginner?

Answer: Start by incorporating more whole, plant-based foods into your meals, such as vegetables, fruits, legumes, nuts, and seeds. Gradually reduce your intake of processed and animal-based foods to align with the diet's principles.

8. How do I know if I'm getting all the nutrients I need on this diet?

Answer: Dr. Li's diet includes nutrient-dense foods that provide essential vitamins, minerals, fiber, and healthy fats. If you're concerned, consider tracking your meals and discussing your diet with a nutritionist to ensure you're getting everything you need.

9. Can I eat snacks on Dr. Li's diet?

Answer: Yes! Dr. Li's diet encourages healthy snacks such as fruits, nuts, seeds, hummus with veggies, or whole-grain crackers. These snacks are nourishing and align with the diet's principles.

10. How do I handle cravings for junk food or processed snacks?

Answer: Cravings can be reduced by choosing healthy, satisfying alternatives, such as roasted nuts, dark chocolate, or fruit. Ensuring that your meals are balanced with enough fiber and protein will help curb unhealthy cravings.

11. How can I make my meals taste flavorful without using added sugars or artificial flavorings?

Answer: Use natural herbs, spices, garlic, onion, lemon, and fresh seasonings to enhance flavor. Ingredients like nutritional yeast, apple cider vinegar, and tahini can add depth to your meals without compromising the diet's principles.

12. Is Dr. Li's diet good for weight loss?

Answer: Yes, Dr. Li's diet promotes whole foods and minimizes processed ingredients, which can naturally lead to weight loss over time. The diet focuses on nutrient-dense foods that keep you satisfied while promoting overall health.

13. How do I know if Dr. Li's diet is right for me?

Answer: If you're looking to improve your overall health, boost energy levels, and prevent or manage chronic disease, Dr. Li's diet may be a great fit. It's a long-term lifestyle change rather than a quick-fix diet.

14. Can I still eat out at restaurants on Dr. Li's diet?

Answer: Yes! Many restaurants offer plant-based options. You can choose dishes that align with the diet, like salads, grilled vegetables, grain bowls, and plant-based proteins. Don't hesitate to ask for modifications, like dressing on the side or no added sugar.

15. How can I stick to Dr. Li's diet if I'm traveling or on vacation?

Answer: Plan ahead by looking up healthy food options in the area. Bring along portable snacks like nuts, fruits, or protein bars. Stick to whole food options, and remember that it's okay to indulge occasionally, but aim to stay true to the diet as much as possible.

16. What are some easy meal ideas to get started with Dr. Li's diet?

Answer: Start with simple meals like quinoa bowls with roasted veggies, salads with leafy greens and legumes, overnight oats with fruit, or stir-fries with tofu and vegetables. These meals are easy to prepare, nutrient-dense, and align with the diet's principles.

17. Can I have desserts on Dr. Li's diet?

Answer: Yes, you can enjoy naturally sweetened desserts like fruit salads, chia pudding, or almond flour-based treats. Focus on using natural sweeteners like dates or maple syrup in moderation.

18. How can I maintain Dr. Li's diet during the holidays or special occasions?

Answer: Plan ahead by bringing your own plant-based dishes to gatherings or requesting modifications to traditional recipes. Stay mindful of portion sizes and remember that one meal won't derail your progress.

19. How long will it take to see results from Dr. Li's diet?

Answer: Results vary depending on individual health conditions and adherence to the diet. You may start feeling better and noticing improvements in energy and digestion within a few weeks. Long-term benefits, such as better heart health and reduced inflammation, can take months.

20. Can Dr. Li's diet help prevent or manage chronic conditions?

Answer: Yes, Dr. Li's diet is designed to support health at the cellular level, boost angiogenesis, and support the microbiome, which can help manage or prevent chronic diseases like heart disease, diabetes, and inflammation-related conditions.

Made in the USA
Monee, IL
15 July 2025